POCKET GUIDE TO
CHINESE PATENT MEDICINES

BY BILL SCHOENBART, L.Ac.

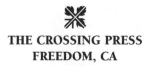

THE CROSSING PRESS
FREEDOM, CA

For information on bulk purchases or group discounts for this and
other Crossing Press titles, please contact our Special Sales Manager
at 800/777-1048.

Visit our Web site on the Internet: www.crossingpress.com

Library of Congress Cataloging-in-Publication Data

Schoenbart, Bill.
    Pocket guide to Chinese patent medicines / by Bill
Schoenbart.
        p. cm. -- (The Crossing Press pocket series)
    Includes bibliographical references.
    ISBN 0-89594-978-4
    1. Herbs -- Therapeutic use -- Handbooks, manuals, etc. 2.
Medicine, Chinese -- Handbooks, manuals, etc. 3. Patent medicines -- Handbooks, manuals, etc. I. Title. II. Title: Chinese
patent medicines III. Series.
    RM666.H33 S366 1999
    615'.321' 0951--dc21   98-47925
                                                            CIP

Disclaimer

This book is for educational purposes only. Patent remedies are normally used as first aid or as a supplement to promote wellness. In no way should they substitute for professional medical treatment. Pregnant women should seek the guidance of a qualified health care practitioner before taking any supplement or herbal medicine. Herbs can have a stronger effect on children, the elderly, or those who are debilitated, so dosages should be decreased in these cases. Children under one year old should not be given herbal medicine without the advice of a practitioner experienced in pediatrics.

Herbal remedies are exceptionally safe, especially when compared to pharmaceutical drugs. However, there is always the possibility of an individual allergic reaction. An inexperienced user may also misdiagnose a condition and select a remedy that is inappropriate. In all cases, discontinue using a patent medicine if you experience a worsening of symptoms or any physical discomfort. If there is any doubt at all, it is best to avoid taking an herbal formula. The best way to use herbal medicine is under the guidance of a qualified health care practitioner.

Contents

Contents

Introduction to Chinese Patent Medicines

It's a familiar scenario: Seemingly out of the blue, a family member starts to feel tired and run-down. Over the next few days, she may develop a sore throat that gradually gets worse. There could be some nasal congestion that spreads into the lungs or sinuses. Over-the-counter remedies may help suppress the symptoms, but they don't affect the duration of the illness, and some can even have dangerous side effects. For example, aspirin can cause stomach ulcers, and acetaminophen can cause liver damage. Often, a sinus infection or bronchitis will develop; a visit to the family doctor may lead to a course of antibiotics. With the use of antibiotics, there is always the risk of a chronic yeast infection, gastrointestinal upset, or impaired immunity.

Is there an alternative way to deal with common colds, coughs, and minor injuries? We need only look to the other side of the planet, to the traditional culture of China, where people have been using natural herbal medicines successfully for thousands of years. In China, the above scenario may begin with the same symptoms, but the response is often far different. After an injury, or at the first sign of a cold or flu, Chinese people turn not to strong pharmaceuticals to suppress their symptoms, but to a vast selection of pre-packaged herbal medicines. There are hundreds of Chinese patent remedies available in convenient, easy-to-use forms like pills and liquids, typically sold in glass bottles and packaged in colorful boxes.

In the past, these prepared medicines often had secret ingredients to enable a manufacturer to distinguish their product from the competitors'. This was the Chinese version of securing a "patent" on the product. While this practice has all but disappeared due to government regulation of herbal medicines, the term "patent medicine" is still used in Western countries to describe pre-packaged over-the-counter Chinese herbal formulas.

Many of these conveniently packaged herbal remedies are intended to treat easily diagnosed, acute, self-limiting conditions like the common cold, coughs, and minor injuries. For example, in the case described above, a person in China might select a remedy formulated to help the body fight off a cold, such as Gan Mao Ling ("gahn maow ling") or Yin Qiao Jie Du Pian ("yin chaow jyeh doo pyen"). If used early enough in the course of a cold or flu, these inexpensive herbal pills will often stop the illness in its tracks. If there is accompanying nasal or sinus congestion, one could also use an herbal decongestant like Bi Yan Pian ("bee yahn pyen") or Chuan Xiong Cha Tiao Wan ("chwahn shuhng chah tyow wahn"). If the cold spreads to the lungs, a cough remedy like Pinellia Root Teapills or Er Chen Wan ("uhr chen wahn") will usually clear the lungs. With the prompt application of herbal patent remedies, it is often possible to halt the progress of a simple cold or other illness before it becomes a more serious condition requiring drug therapy.

FORMS OF PATENT MEDICINES

Pills: This is the most common form of patent medicines. The usual procedure is to boil an herbal formula until it becomes highly concentrated. This thickened mass is then rolled into tiny balls that are air-dried with a protective glaze. These are then typically placed in glass bottles and sealed with a cork and a plastic cap. This format has a number of advantages. The small size makes the pills easy to swallow, and the fact that they are already extracted in water makes them easy to assimilate. In Chinese, this type of pill is called wan ("wahn"), so it is common for a patent medicine's name to end with this word. For example, Six Flavor Rehmannia Pills are known as Liu Wei Di Huang Wan. Liu Wei means "six flavors," Di Huang means "Rehmannia root," and Wan means "round pill."

Tablets: This is another popular method of administering herbs. Known in Chinese as pian ("pyen"), these are either flattened discs or sugar-coated tablets (i.e., the shape of a few popular brands of coated candies). The disc-shaped tablets are a little difficult for some people to swallow, but the coated tablets are very easy to swallow. Children will have less difficulty taking this form of tablet.[1] An example of this format would be the remedy known as Bi Yan Pian ("nose inflammation tablets").

Granules or Instant Teas: Granules are an excellent way to give herbs to children. They are made by boiling down the herbs into a concentrated decoction and then crystallizing the liquid on a heated surface. They can be stirred into hot water to make a refreshing tea. For children who tend to balk at taking medicines, they can be hidden in foods like apple sauce. These instant teas are known as chong ji ("chung jee"). An example from this book would be Luo Han Guo Chong Ji.

Liquids: There are a variety of liquid formats for patent remedies. Ginseng extracts are commonly sold in small vials mixed with honey. This is the form that many Americans have seen. There are also herbal wines, syrups, and preserved

---

[1]Children should never be told these are candy. Herbs, like all medications, should be kept securely out of the reach of children.

liquid extracts. These are readily absorbed and are usually pleasant tasting. Some examples from this book are Extractum Astragali and Tang Kwei Gin.

Powders: Some herbs work better in their raw form, or they contain volatile ingredients that will be destroyed by cooking. Medicines in this form are sold loose in glass bottles or in gelatin capsules. Examples of medicines in this form would be Sai Mei An or Yunnan Pai Yao.

Liniments or Medicated Oils: With rare exceptions, herbs in this form are meant for external use only. They are typically used for bruises, fractures, or sprains. An example would be Zheng Gu Shui, which translates as "setting bone liquid."

Plasters: These are self-adhering pieces of cloth or plastic that have their adhesive saturated with an herbal concentrate. They are applied directly to the skin, and the medicinal qualities of the herbs penetrate the area to relieve pain. An example of this effective type of remedy would be Die Da Zhi Tong Gao (Plaster for Bruise and Analgesic).

DOSAGE

A recommended dosage will be printed on the bottle by the manufacturer. Unless instructed otherwise by a practitioner, it is best to avoid exceeding this amount. Don't be alarmed if a dosage sounds very large; for example, a common dosage is 8 pills, 3 times per day. In most cases, these will be tiny round pills that are very easy to swallow. In fact, it is much easier to swallow eight small pills at once than one large pill or capsule. It is also important to remember that because patent remedies are made from herbs, it is necessary to take a larger dose than one would take of powerful, concentrated drugs.

When giving herbs to children, a good rule of thumb is Clark's Rule, a standard method of determining drug doses according to body weight. Assuming that the average adult weighs 150 pounds, the child's weight is divided by 150 to determine the reduction in dosage. For example, if the child weighs 50 pounds, the dose would be 50/150, or 1/3 the adult dose. If the adult dose is 15 pills, the 50-pound child would take 5 pills. Children less than one year of age, elderly, or weak individuals should not be given herbal medicine unless on the advice of a qualified health care practitioner.

SAFETY ISSUES

While Chinese patent medicines are normally a safe and convenient way to ingest healing herbs, there are some important safety issues to consider. Of greatest concern is the possible presence of heavy metals and pharmaceutical drugs in these products. These adulterants can make their way into a formula in a number of ways:

1. In China and Taiwan, herbs and drugs are intentionally mixed in certain products to achieve a synergistic action. Sometimes the drugs are listed on the label, but sometimes they are omitted.

2. Unauthorized or irresponsible factories might use polluted water containing heavy metals in the decoction process. These same factories might also skip crucial quality control procedures designed to detect the presence of pesticides in the herbs.

3. Some formulas intentionally include minerals containing heavy metals to achieve their therapeutic effect. This practice may have been acceptable in pre-industrial times, when heavy metal exposure was minimal. However, in modern times people already have overly high exposures

due to industrial pollution, and any further exposure is unacceptable.

Fortunately, all of these concerns can be addressed to ensure that your use of Chinese patent medicines is a safe and healing experience. The most important thing to know is that there are manufacturers in China that *never* use drugs, artificial coloring, or any additives or contaminants in their products. I recommend that you use medicines manufactured at facilities that adhere to Good Manufacturing Practices (G.M.P.), which are quality standards followed by Western pharmaceutical companies. One of the best examples of a G.M.P. facility in China is the Lanzhou Foci Herb Company. They have exceptionally high standards of quality control in all steps of the manufacturing process. Lanzhou Foci, like other good manufacturers, attempts to purchase all their raw herbs from farmers who avoid the use of pesticides, and will test the herbs, in their raw state and after they are extracted, for the presence of pesticides. They also filter all their water, and they test their finished products for heavy metals and molds.

There are about ten G.M.P. factories in China, and the products of other G.M.P. facilities are reviewed in this book—Qi Xing and Pangaoshou, for example, are also G.M.P. facilities. Most of the patents reviewed in this book are made by Lanzhou Foci or Plum Flower. In my experience, these are reliable lines with high standards of quality; they are by no means the only good lines of patent medicine. While Plum Flower brand—which is guaranteed to have no dyes, pharmaceuticals, or heavy metals—is only available from Mayway Corporation, Lanzhou Foci products can be found in Chinatowns and herb stores all over the world. Unfortunately, counterfeit versions of high-quality products are also very common: these use a similar color, design, or name. In the case of Lanzhou Foci, look for their *full* name on the label.

The Food and Drug branch of the California Department of Health Services has recently investigated the issue of heavy metals and pharmaceuticals in Chinese patent medicines. Over 600 products were tested, and the results of 260 of the product tests are described in a report entitled *Compendium of Asian Patent Medicines*. As of this writing (May, 1998) the project is not complete, but all pertinent information is included in the description of any products that might be affected by contamination. In these cases, an uncontaminated product will be recommended.

HOW TO GET STARTED

In China, people usually receive a patent medicine at a hospital or an herbal pharmacy. In either case, they are likely to have been accurately diagnosed before they select a remedy. In Western countries, licensed acupuncturists are the practitioners most likely to be thoroughly trained in the traditional Chinese diagnostic system. This is especially true in California, where all acupuncturists are required to be proficient in herbal medicine. In other states, practitioners can demonstrate their proficiency by passing an herbal exam given by the National Commission for the Certification of Acupuncturists. It is highly recommended that you consult with a qualified practitioner of Chinese herbal medicine before attempting to use patent remedies. If you are interested in becoming a practitioner of acupuncture and herbal medicine, the rigorous training takes from three to four years and involves both academic studies and clinical practice. Names of schools can be obtained from the organizations listed at the end of the book.

HOW TO USE THIS BOOK

The remedies are organized according to organ systems and diagnostic categories. Some formulas could easily be included in several categories. In these cases the formula is listed under its most common usage. Within each category, the medicines are placed in alphabetical order. Each medicine is described in the following format:

Title: The name of the remedy, as it appears on the box. Example: Shu Gan Wan

Pronunciation and translation: To aid in pronunciation, the formula's name will be spelled phonetically. This will be followed by a literal translation of the name. Example: "shoo gahn wahn"—"soothe liver pill"

Indications: This is the range of symptoms for which the formula is indicated, though not all symptoms are necessarily present at the same time. Example: Digestive disorders that become worse under stress; abdominal distention and pain, nausea, belching, poor appetite, gas, and loose stools.

Ingredients: Each ingredient in the formula is listed. Herbs are given their Latin botanical name, along with their Chinese name in parentheses. Example:

Bupleurum chinense root (Chai Hu)
Curcuma longa rhizome (Jiang Huang)

Description: This section will explain the action, ingredients, and Chinese and Western diagnostic categories of the formula. Lifestyle and dietary suggestions might also be included. Example: "When this pattern occurs, it is important to use a formula that soothes the Liver and also resolves the digestive difficulties. This remedy addresses both areas. While this remedy will usually resolve the imbalance, it is important to reduce the sources of stress that cause this pattern. It is helpful to avoid alcohol and high-fat foods, as well as eating on the run or while upset."

Dosage: The recommended dosage as provided by the manufacturer is given. In some cases of acute ailments, a practitioner might increase the dosage. On the other hand, dosages are decreased for children, elderly, or weak individuals. Example: 8 pills, 3 times per day

Manufacturer: Although there are often many manufacturers of a given remedy, the recommended one is listed. This is very important, since some manufacturers have very high standards of purity. They avoid using artificial coloring and pharmaceuticals, and they test for heavy metals and pesticides. Example: Lanzhou Foci

Warnings and contraindications: This will explain when the remedy is inappropriate or dangerous. Example: Do not use during pregnancy.

Traditional Chinese herbal medicine is a fascinating and intricate system of healing. While it can take a lifetime to become an expert at creating herbal formulas, studying the patent remedies provides the layperson with an excellent introduction to this ancient practice. It is my hope that this pocket guide will kindle a lifelong interest in the healing properties of herbs. Whether they come from China or your own yard, medicinal herbs are among nature's great gifts to humanity. Used wisely and with respect, they can greatly enhance the quality of your life.

Bill Schoenbart, L.Ac.

The Philosophy of Chinese Herbal Medicine

Many patent remedies are based on herbal formulas that have been in use for more than two thousand years. These formulas have gone through extensive human trials over a long period, and a skilled practitioner of herbal medicine can use them to treat extremely subtle and complex chronic conditions. To determine which formula to use, a diagnosis is made according to ancient principles that were developed by the Taoist sages, who were especially keen observers of the human body and its relationship to nature. Their worldview helped to shape the theoretical foundation for Chinese medicine as it is practiced today.

YIN AND YANG IN NATURE AND THE HUMAN BODY

Through patient observation of the forces of nature, the Taoists saw the universe as a unified field, constantly moving and changing while maintaining its oneness. This constant state of change was explained by the theory of Yin and Yang, which first appeared in written form around 700 B.C. in the *I Ching* ("Book of Changes"). According to this theory, nature expresses itself in a dynamic cycle of polar opposites such as day and night, moisture and dryness, heat and cold, or activity and rest. Yin phenomena are those that exhibit the nurturing qualities of darkness, rest, moisture, cold, and structure. Yang phenomena in turn have energetic qualities such as light, activity, dryness, heat, and function. Everything in nature exhibits varying combinations of Yin and Yang. The morning fog (Yin) is dissipated by the heat of the

Sun (Yang); the forest fire (Yang) is extinguished by the rainstorm (Yin); the darkness of night (Yin) is replaced by the light of day (Yang). In this way, any phenomenon in nature can be understood in relationship to another; one will always be more Yin or Yang than the other.

Since the Taoists believed that everything in the universe is essentially one, they made no distinction between the external forces of nature and the internal processes of the human body. This gave rise to the belief that "the macrocosm exists within the microcosm." In other words, any process or change that can be witnessed in nature can also be seen in the human body. For example, a person who eats cold food (Yin) on a cold, damp day (Yin) will often experience excessive mucus (Yin). Similarly, a person who performs strenuous activity (Yang) on a hot day (Yang) might experience dehydration with a fever (Yang). Some of the traditional diagnoses sound like a weather report, such as "*wind* and *cold* with *dampness*" (a Yin condition); or "a deficiency of *moisture* leading to *fire*" (a Yang pattern). These diagnostic descriptions illustrate the principle that the human body experiences the same fluctuations of Yin and Yang as the environment.

The internal organs also have their own balance of Yin and Yang. Yin qualities tend to be nourishing, cooling, building, relaxing, and related to the structure of the organs. Yang qualities tend to be energizing, warming, consuming, stimulating, and related to the functional activity of the organs. The organs in Chinese medicine are the Heart, Lungs, Spleen, Liver, Kidneys, Pericardium, Large Intestine, Small Intestine, Gall Bladder, Stomach, and Urinary Bladder. Each organ possesses functions that closely parallel those of its Western counterpart, but they also have additional functions that are unique to Chinese medicine. Since all the organs have Yin and Yang aspects, it is possible to monitor and adjust the levels of Yin and Yang in all parts of the body, maintaining a high level of vitality and preventing imbalances which manifest as disease. This is achieved not only with herbal medicine, but with changes in diet and lifestyle as well. In this way, the observations of the ancient Taoists have practical applications in the modern world in our quest for wellness and preventive health care.

THE VITAL SUBSTANCES: QI AND BLOOD

In addition to Yin and Yang, traditional Chinese medicine also uses the concepts of two vital substances: Qi ("chee") and Blood. Although Qi plays a central role in traditional Chinese medicine, it is extremely difficult to define. Existing somewhere between matter and energy, Qi has the qualities of both. It has substance without structure, and it possesses energetic qualities, but can't be measured. It is the fundamental power underlying all the activities of nature, as well as the vital life force of the human body.

It is easiest to understand Qi in terms of its functions and activities, where it is readily perceived. For example, the force of a thunderstorm can be understood in terms of its Qi; similarly, the strength of the digestive organs can be evaluated in relation to their Qi. In the storm, the power of the Qi can be observed in the fallen trees and buildings in the storm's aftermath; in the body, the strength of digestive Qi can be evaluated by the appetite and how the body assimilates nutrition.

Although there are many types of specialized Qi in the body, all varieties share some basic functions. Qi is responsible for transforming one type of substance into another.

The Qi of digestion (Spleen Qi) transforms food into usable energy and blood; Kidney Qi transforms fluids into pure essence and waste water; Lung Qi transforms air into the energy to sustain life. Qi is also responsible for protecting the body from attacks by external pathogens. If the Qi is weak, a person may get frequent colds and other illnesses. Qi keeps organs in their proper place, blood within the vessels, and body fluids inside the body. Deficiency of Qi can lead to sagging organs (prolapse), bleeding disorders, and excessive sweating or urination. The Yang Qi of the Kidney is responsible for keeping the entire body warm; when it is deficient, a person can experience chronic cold extremities and decreased function in all activities that require warmth, such as digestion.

Blood has some parallels to its Western counterpart, such as its function of circulating through the body and nourishing the organs. However, it also has some very subtle functions in Chinese medicine, such as providing a substantial foundation for the mind and lending sensitivity to the sensory organs. It is closely aligned with Qi, having a complementary relationship with it. There is a saying, "Blood is the mother of Qi, and Qi is the leader of Blood." This refers to the fact that without Blood, there is no fundamental nutritional basis for Qi; without Qi, there would be no ability to form or circulate Blood, and it would fail to stay within the vessels. The two are also considered to flow together through the body.

The main function of Blood is to circulate throughout the body, providing nourishment and moisture to the organs, skin, muscles, and tendons. If it is deficient, there can be symptoms such as dry skin and hair, inflexible tendons, or various emotional and reproductive imbalances, depending on which organs are involved. If it is stagnant, there will be sharp pain at the site of stagnation. If there is heat in the Blood, there can be irritability and skin rashes. Since Qi and Blood are so closely related, a deficiency or stagnation of one of the substances will often lead to the same imbalance in the other.

CAUSES OF IMBALANCE: THE SIX PATHOGENIC FACTORS

Another important concept that the Taoists contributed to Chinese medicine is the realization that the interior of the human body works in much the same way as the world outside the body. Through careful observation, they noted that the body could develop its own "weather patterns," often in response to the external environment. These six patterns, known as pathogenic factors, are *wind, cold, heat, dampness, dryness,* and *summer heat.*

The pathogenic factor of *wind* is considered to be the major cause of illness in traditional diagnosis. It readily combines with other pathogens, giving rise to syndromes like *wind cold, wind heat,* and *wind dampness.* It possesses qualities of the wind as seen in nature, appearing without warning and constantly changing. It is considered to be a Yang pathogenic factor, especially attacking the upper body, head, throat, and eyes. *Wind* causes things to move, so it is usually involved when there is twitching, spasms, and shaking. The organ most often affected by external *wind* is the Lung; internal *wind* is most commonly related to an imbalance in the Liver.

Cold is considered to be a Yin pathogenic factor. Its nature is to slow things down, causing tightness, stagnation, contraction, and an impairment in circulation. Externally, it can attack the skin, muscles, and Lungs. Internally, it can cause an impairment in the normal functions of the Spleen, Stomach, and Kidneys.

Heat, or *fire*, is a Yang pathogenic factor. As in nature, *heat* causes expansion and increased activity. When out of balance, it can lead to irritability, fever, and inflammatory conditions. By its nature it rises up, manifesting as a red face and eyes, dizziness, anger, and sore throat. It tends to deplete the body fluids, leading to thirst, constipation, and dark urine. Since it can produce *wind*, it can lead to spasmodic movement.

In nature, dampness soaks the ground and everything that comes in contact with it, creating a stagnant situation. Once something becomes damp, especially in wet weather, it can take a long time to dry out again. The Yin pathogenic influence of *dampness* has similar qualities: it is persistent, heavy, and it can be difficult to resolve. A person who spends a lot of time in the rain, lives in a damp environment, or sleeps on the ground can be more susceptible to an attack of external *dampness*. Similarly, a person who eats large amounts of ice cream, cold foods, cold drinks, greasy foods, and sweets is prone to imbalances of internal *dampness*. In general, symptoms of *dampness* in the body include water retention (edema), swelling, feelings of heaviness, coughing or vomiting phlegm, and wet skin eruptions. When *dampness* combines with *heat*, the condition of *damp heat* develops. This can cause a variety of symptoms such as dark, burning urine, sticky, foul-smelling stools, yellow vaginal discharges, and jaundice.

Dryness is a Yang pathogenic influence. As in nature, its influence on the body is drying and astringent. It can easily deplete the body fluids, causing constipation, concentrated urine, dryness in the throat and nose, thirst, dry skin, and dry cough. It typically enters the body through the nose and mouth, quickly affecting the Lungs.

Summer heat is a Yang pathogenic influence that usually occurs in the heat and humidity of summer. It affects the head area, causing thirst, red face, and headache; a person will tend to lie down with the limbs spread out. The excessive sweating also causes the urine to be dark and concentrated, and there can be a depletion of the body's Yin. The extreme *heat* also affects the heart, leading to restlessness or coma in severe cases like sunstroke. When it combines with *dampness* due to humidity and over-consumption of soft drinks, the Spleen is also affected. This leads to a loss of appetite, nausea, vomiting, diarrhea, and fatigue.

DIAGNOSIS AND TREATMENT

Before prescribing an herbal formula, a trained practitioner of Chinese medicine will look for the presence of the six pathogenic factors and assess the levels of Yin, Yang, Qi, and Blood in the organs. This is done by taking an accurate history of the person's symptoms and performing a tongue and pulse diagnosis.

The condition of each of the internal organs can be determined by looking at the tongue and feeling the pulse. Different areas of the tongue represent the different organ systems. The color and shape of the tongue and its coating in each area reflects the condition of the corresponding organ. If the tongue itself is bright red this indicates *heat*, while a pale color indicates *cold*. Similarly, a yellow tongue coating is a sign of *heat*, while a white tongue coating is a sign of *cold*. For example, the back of the tongue is the area that corresponds to the Urinary Bladder. If that area has a thick and greasy yellow coating, a practitioner might suspect a bladder infection ("*damp heat* in the Urinary Bladder").

The pulses on the wrists would then be palpated. If the pulse corresponding to the Bladder is rapid and strong and has a "rolling" feeling, the physician would have further support for the diagnosis of *damp heat*. Finally, the patient's symptoms of dark, burning urine and abdominal pain would provide enough evidence to confirm the diagnosis.

Once an accurate diagnosis is made, the practitioner will select an herbal formula that has a long history of successfully treating that particular condition. Herbal formulas are organized according to traditional diagnostic categories and the organ systems that are to be treated. Each formula in a diagnostic category has a particular focus. For example, within the category of formulas that treat the common cold (*wind*), there are two subcategories: formulas that treat *cold*-type conditions (*wind cold*) and formulas that treat *heat*-type conditions (*wind heat*). Within those subcategories, some formulas might focus on symptoms that are more predominant, such as a dry cough or a sore throat. To further discriminate, certain ingredients may be added or eliminated to alter the effects of a formula.

Chinese herbal formulas are organized according to a hierarchy. The chief herb in a formula is the most important ingredient, having the most direct effect on the primary disorder. The deputy herb either augments the chief herb in treating the principal pattern, or it addresses another set of symptoms. The assistant herb can help the chief and deputy in their functions, or it can moderate their effects. Finally, the envoy herb can direct the actions of the formula to a certain area of the body, or it can act to detoxify or harmonize the other ingredients. This method of organizing formulas is quite complex, and there are differing opinions among experts over which herbs occupy various positions in the hierarchy. However, the end result is a system of diagnosis and treatment that has withstood the test of time due to its high rate of success in treating the full range of human ailments.

As you can imagine, traditional Chinese diagnosis is a very subtle and intricate process that can take an entire lifetime to master. For this reason, the beginning student of Chinese herbal medicine will have an easier time by first learning how to use the patent medicines. They often have the same ingredients as traditional formulas, but they are easier and more convenient to use. They are also less likely to cause a problem if they are used incorrectly, since they are not as strong as bulk herbs boiled in decoctions. However, it is still preferable to receive a competent diagnosis from a trained practitioner before attempting to use the patent medicines. Your learning experience will be enhanced and you are more likely to feel the full benefits of an accurately prescribed herbal formula.

Remedies for the Circulatory System

Dan Shen Yin Wan
Pronunciation and translation: "dahn shen yin wahn"—
"red sage drink pill"
Indications: Pain from angina

Ingredients:
Salvia miltiorrhiza root (Dan Shen)
Santalum album wood (Tan Xiang)
Amomum villosum fruit (Sha Ren)

Description: Coronary artery disease and angina pain have
become far too common in modern industrialized countries.
There are a number of herbs in Chinese medicine that exert
a powerful effect on the heart, clearing cholesterol deposits
and increasing efficiency of the heart muscle. These herbs
are a valuable supplement to Western medical treatment,
and they are among the great gifts of the contemporary
practice of Chinese herbal medicine.

The most important herb for treating heart disease is
Salvia miltiorrhiza (Dan Shen). The root of this member of
the Sage genus contains constituents that have remarkable
healing effects on the heart muscle and coronary arteries. In
fact, it is so effective that heart attack patients in China receive
an intravenous drip of a sterile Salvia extract when they arrive
at the emergency room. It has multiple actions, reducing cholesterol levels, relieving pain and anxiety, and promoting a
more rapid recovery. It dilates the coronary artery, adjusts the
heart rate, inhibits coagulation, and increases blood flow to

the heart muscle. Numerous research studies, both with the whole herb and with this patent medicine, have demonstrated the effectiveness of Salvia. In one study, 80 percent of the patients who received Dan Shen experienced a remission of angina pain and chest fullness. EKG readings showed an improvement in up to 50 percent of the patients after one month; a higher percentage showed improvement after one year.

Of course, it is essential for a person with heart disease to make radical lifestyle improvements, including diet and exercise programs supervised by their physician. No amount of medicine, whether pharmaceutical or herbal, will be successful in the long term without making these important adjustments.

Dosage: 8 pills, 3 times per day

Manufacturer: Plum Flower

Warnings and contraindications: This condition should *always* be treated by a physician; failure to receive prompt medical care increases the risk of sudden death or disability. Attempting to self-treat such a condition is extremely unwise, since even a one-hour delay in receiving medical treatment can be a fatal error if the blockage worsens and leads to a heart attack. The only appropriate use for this remedy in the event of a heart attack would be while waiting for an ambulance to arrive. For chronic heart problems, this remedy should *only* be used under the supervision of a physician.

Hawthorn Fat-Reducing Tablets

Indications: High cholesterol, angina, obesity

Ingredients:

Crataegus pinnatifida fruit (Shan Zha)

Description: Hawthorn fruit has been traditionally used in Chinese medicine for "food stagnation," the prolonged retention of food in the stomach. It is especially appropriate when the indigestion is caused by overeating fatty foods, due to its ability to break down fats. This fat-digesting action also makes Hawthorn useful in bringing down high cholesterol levels and reducing fat deposits in the body. A popular dieting tea, known as Bojenmi, is simply a mixture of tea leaves and Hawthorn.

The cardiac activity of this incredibly useful herb is not limited to its ability to break down cholesterol deposits. Hawthorn lowers blood pressure slowly and persistently, with the effect lasting for approximately three hours. It also dilates blood vessels and increases blood flow to the coronary artery. It is quite safe and can be used for extended periods of time.

Dosage: 1–2 tablets, 3 times per day

Manufacturer: Sanming Pharmaceutical Manufactory

Warnings and contraindications: Do not attempt self-treatment for heart disease. If you are taking cardiac drugs, consult your physician before using Hawthorn, as it may increase the effect of the drugs.

While this product showed no traces of contamination when tested, it does contain some sugar. Hawthorn is also commonly used in Western herbalism, so there is a wide range of high-quality solid and liquid extracts available from health food and herb stores.

Remedies for the Digestive System

Huang Lian Su

Pronunciation and translation: "hwahng lyan soo"— "coptis extract"

Indications: Diarrhea or dysentery due to bacterial infection

Ingredients:

Berberine extracted from Coptis chinensis rhizome (Huang Lian)

Description: This patent medicine walks the line between herbs and drugs. The word "Su" refers to a specific constituent isolated from an herb. In this case, the constituent is berberine, a bright yellow-colored alkaloid that is also present in Western herbs like Goldenseal and Oregon Grape. Berberine is a broad spectrum antibacterial and antiparasitic, making this remedy extremely useful for the treatment of "traveler's diarrhea." On their journeys to India, China, Africa, and Central America, travelers often send postcards containing glowing references to "those little yellow pills." For best results, it is advised to combine Huang Lian Su with a remedy that normalizes intestinal function, such as Mu Xiang Shun Qi Wan (see p. 30).

Huang Lian (Coptis chinensis) also has strong inhibitory effects on the bacteria that cause streptococcal and staphylococcal infections, pneumonia, and dysentery. Studies have shown it to be as effective as sulfa drugs in treating dysentery, without the serious side effects. Clinical trials have also proved it to be effective in treating influenza, pertussis (whooping cough), typhoid fever, tuberculosis, scarlet fever, and diphtheria. In China herbal medicine is used with great success to treat serious disease as well as minor ailments.

Dosage: 2 pills, 3 times per day

Manufacturer: Min-Kang Drug Manufactory

Warnings and contraindications: Not appropriate for diarrhea from non-bacterial causes, such as chronic indigestion, stomach flu, or overeating.

This remedy is for acute infections only. Do not use for more than a week or two. For best results, it is advisable to replenish intestinal flora (by taking acidophilus or bifidus supplements) after using this remedy. If diarrhea persists, see your health care practitioner.

Huo Xiang Zheng Qi Wan; Lophanthus Antifebrile

Pronunciation and translation: "haw shahng jung chee wahn"—"agastache Qi-normalizing pills"

Indications: Stomach flu, nausea, vomiting, diarrhea, sticky stools

Ingredients:

Agastache rugosa plant (Huo Xiang)

Angelica dahurica root (Bai Zhi)

Areca acacia husk (Da Fu Pi)

Perilla frutescens leaf (Zi Su Ye)

Poria cocos fungus (Fu Ling)

Glycyrrhiza uralensis root (Gan Cao)

Atractylodes macrocephala root (Bai Zhu)

Magnolia officinalis bark (Hou Po)

Platycodon grandiflorum root (Jie Geng)

Citrus reticulata peel (Chen Pi)

Description: This is one of the best patent remedies for stomach flu. In traditional Chinese herbal medicine, it is indicated for a specific pattern that often occurs in the summer, with symptoms of nausea, vomiting, diarrhea, gas, headache, and sometimes fever and chills. When the symptoms are mild, it works quite well on its own, often bringing relief after just one dose. When symptoms are more severe, it is best to take it along with Gan Mao Ling (see p. 76) to enhance its ability to ward off the external pathogenic influence.

Dosage: 10 pills, 3 times per day

Manufacturer: Lanzhou Foci

Warnings and contraindications: This formula has some herbs that are drying. Do not use it when the signs of *heat* are prominent, such as a dry mouth, thirst, or high fever.

Mu Xiang Shun Qi Wan

Pronunciation and translation: "moo shahng shuhn chee wahn"—"saussurea Qi-regulating pills"

Indications: Food stagnation, indigestion, diarrhea, and intestinal gas

Ingredients:

Saussurea lappa root (Mu Xiang)

Alpinia katsumadai seed (Cao Dou Kou)

Atractylodes lancea rhizome (Cang Zhu)

Zingiberis officinalis rhizome (Sheng Jiang)

Citrus reticulata peel (Chen Pi)

Citrus reticulata green peel (Qing Pi)

Poria cocos fungus (Fu Ling)

Bupleurum chinense root (Chai Hu)

Magnolia officinalis bark (Hou Po)

Areca catechu seed (Bing Lang)

Poncirus trifoliata fruit (Zhi Shi)

Lindera strychnifolia root (Wu Yao)

Raphanus sativa seed (Lai Fu Zi)

Crataegus pinnatifida fruit (Shan Zha)

Fermentata medicinalis mass (Shen Qu)

Hordeum vulgare sprout (Mai Ya)

Glycyrrhiza uralensis root (Gan Cao)

Description: This formula relieves stagnation in the gastrointestinal tract, with symptoms such as fullness in the abdominal area, distention, gas, diarrhea, and a sensation of food sitting in the stomach without being digested. The chief herb in the remedy is Saussurea (Mu Xiang), which has the ability to reduce pain and fullness in the stomach and intestines caused by stagnation of Qi (vital energy). To enhance its effect of moving energy in the digestive tract, it is combined with other Qi-moving herbs, including Alpinia, Green Citrus, Magnolia, Areca, Poncirus, and Lindera. To alleviate the problem of food stagnating in the stomach, the following herbs are added: Raphanus (Radish seed), Crataegus (Hawthorn), Hordeum (Barley sprout), and a mixture of fermented grains and herbs (Shen Qu). The end result of this combination is a strong synergistic action that promotes peristalsis, relieves pain and fullness, and restores normal digestive function.

Mu Xiang Shun Qi Wan is especially helpful in treating traveler's diarrhea when combined with Huang Lian Su (see p. 28). The latter kills the pathogens responsible for the diarrhea, while the former restores normal intestinal function. Because the combination of these two remedies is remarkably effective, it is highly recommended to include them in home first aid or travel kits.

Dosage: 8 pills, 3 times per day

Manufacturer: Lanzhou Foci

Warnings and contraindications: If diarrhea persists, see your health care practitioner. In all cases of diarrhea, it is important to drink plenty of fluids to avoid dehydration. In severe or prolonged cases, I.V. fluids and electrolytes may need to be administered.

Peach Kernel Pills; Run Chang Wan

Pronunciation and translation: "ruhn chahng wahn"— "moisten intestines pills"

Indications: Constipation due to excess heat or dryness in the intestines

Ingredients:

Cannabis sativa seed (Huo Ma Ren)

Prunus persica seed (Tao Ren)

Cistanche salsa plant (Rou Cong Rong)

Angelica sinensis root (Dang Gui)

Rheum palmatum rhizome (Da Huang)

Description: This is a rather simple treatment for constipation. *Heat* or *dryness* lodging in the intestines can dry out the intestinal walls and the stools, preventing smooth movement of the bowels. This formula lubricates the intestines with Yin-nourishing oily seeds like Cannabis and Prunus (Peach pit). Cistanche is included for its ability to strengthen the Yang-eliminative power of the bowel, while Dang Gui nourishes the Blood and moistens the walls of the intestine. Finally, Rhubarb rhizome (Da Huang) has strong purgative qualities, effectively moving the bowels as well as clearing the *heat* that causes constipation.

Dosage: 4–8 pills, three times per day
Manufacturer: Lanzhou Foci
Warnings and contraindications: Since Rhubarb is a strong purgative herb, this remedy is for short-term use only. Constipation is usually the result of dietary indiscretions, especially insufficient fiber and fluids. It can often be rectified with a diet high in juicy vegetables, boiled whole grains, sufficient fluids, and high-quality oils like sesame, olive, and flax.

Pill Curing; Kang Ning Wan

Pronunciation and translation: "kahng ning wahn"— "healthy quiet pills"
Indications: Disorders of the stomach such as nausea, vomiting, fullness, acidity, motion sickness, or acid regurgitation

Ingredients:

Gastrodia elata rhizome (Tian Ma)
Angelica dahurica root (Bai Zhi)
Chrysanthemum morifolium flower (Ju Hua)
Mentha haplocalyx plant (Bo He)
Pueraria lobata root (Ge Gen)
Trichosanthes kirilowii root (Tian Hua Fen)
Atractylodes lancea rhizome (Cang Zhu)
Coix lachryma-jobi seed (Yi Yi Ren)
Poria cocos fungus (Fu Ling)
Saussurea lappa root (Mu Xiang)
Magnolia officinalis bark (Hou Po)
Citrus erythrocarpa peel (Ju Hong)
Agastache rugosa plant (Huo Xiang)
Fermentata medicinalis mass (Shen Qu)
Oryza sativa sprout (Gu Ya)

Description: Pill Curing, also known as "Curing Pills," are extremely popular both in China and the West. They can be used for upset stomach due to overeating, weak digestion, or any other cause. For motion sickness, they should be taken 30 to 60 minutes before traveling. To enhance the effect, they can be taken with Ginger in capsules or as a tea, since Ginger has been shown in clinical trials to be more effective than Dramamine in relieving motion sickness. The combination of Ginger and Curing Pills is extremely effective. To treat nausea and vomiting that accompanies a cold or flu, this remedy can be combined with Gan Mao Ling (see p. 76).

Dosage: 1–2 vials, 3 times per day, or as needed.

Each vial is filled with tiny pills, and it is quite easy to wash down a whole vial of pills with water.

Manufacturer: United Pharmaceutical Manufactory; Plum Flower

Warnings and contraindications: Many different manufacturers produce nearly identical versions of this product, and many of these contain artificial food coloring. There is now a dye-free version made by Plum Flower.

Sai Mei An

Pronunciation and translation: "sai may ahn"—"made by Sai Mei An factory"

Indications: Irritation to the stomach lining, gastric or duodenal ulcer without bleeding

Ingredients:

Stalactite mineral (Zhing Ru Shi)

Calcite mineral (Han Shui Shi)

Dryobalanops aromatica crystal [Borneol camphor] (Bing Pian)

Pteria margaritifera shell (Zhen Zhu)
Arca inflata shell (Wa Leng Zi)
Fuligo herbarum (Bai Cao Shuang)
Cyclina sinensis shell (Hai Ge Ke)

Description: Sai Mei An is an interesting combination of powdered minerals and shells that neutralizes excess stomach acid and forms a protective coating on the stomach wall. This protects an ulcer from further irritation from food and acids, allowing it time to heal. Normally the process takes two weeks or more. During this time irritating foods such as coffee and spices should be avoided. An especially effective regimen could include the daily use of Licorice root. This is available in health food stores as Deglycyrrhized Licorice (DGL); clinical studies have shown that it has a high success rate in treating ulcers.

Sai Mei An can also be used topically for mouth ulcers. Simply open a cap and sprinkle some of the powder directly on the ulcer. For *damp*-type skin irritations such as poison ivy/oak rashes, empty a capsule into the palm of your hand. Add a few drops of water, make into a paste with your finger, and apply it to the irritated area. The effect is soothing and cooling due to the Borneol camphor crystals, and the shell powders will help dry out the pustules. For an extra drying effect, the Sai Mei An powder can be mixed with a little French green clay powder before making it into a paste.

Dosage: 3 pills, 3 times per day, one half hour before meals

Manufacturer: Sai Mei An Medicine Factory

Warnings and contraindications: Dark, tar-like stools or vomiting blood can indicate a serious bleeding ulcer. Seek medical attention immediately.

Shen Ling Bai Zhu Pian

Pronunciation and translation: "shen ling bye zhoo pyahn"—"codonopsis, poria, and atractylodes pills"

Indications: Gastro-intestinal problems due to weak digestion, such as loose stools, bloating, and belching

Ingredients:

Codonopsis pilosula root (Dang Shen)

Poria cocos fungus (Fu Ling)

Atractylodes macrocephala rhizome (Bai Zhu)

Platycodon grandiflorum root (Jie Geng)

Dioscorea opposita root (Shan Yao)

Citrus reticulata peel (Chen Pi)

Amomum villosum seed (Sha Ren)

Nelumbo nucifera seed (Lian Zi)

Dolichoris lablab seed (Bai Bian Dou)

Coix lachryma-jobi seed (Yi Yi Ren)

Glycyrrhiza uralensis prepared root (Zhi Gan Cao)

Description: Shen Ling Bai Zhu Pian gets its name from the tonic herbs Dang Shen, Fu Ling, and Bai Zhu. These herbs strengthen the digestive Qi and remove the *damp* intestinal environment that causes diarrhea. The word Pian refers to a pill that is somewhat disc-shaped. In this way, a simple Chinese five-word title lists the main ingredients of the formula and describes the shape of the pill. Unlike Huang Lian Su (see p. 28), which treats diarrhea due to bacterial or parasitic infection, this remedy rectifies diarrhea caused by weakness in the digestive system.

In traditional Chinese diagnosis, the Qi (vital energy) of the Spleen is responsible for proper digestion and assimilation of nutrients. When the Spleen Qi is deficient, the result can be watery diarrhea or undigested food in the stools. Often this will be a chronic condition, caused by an inherited weakness or induced by poor eating habits. This situation is rectified through the use of tonic herbs that strengthen the Qi and thereby improve metabolism. In traditional formulation, some herbs will treat the cause of the problem, which is known as the root. Other herbs will address a specific symptom, known as the branch. Shen Ling Bai Zhu Pian contains herbs that treat both the root cause (Qi deficiency) and the branch symptom (diarrhea), making it effective both in the short and long term. The main herb treating the branch symptom of diarrhea is Lotus seed (Lian Zi), which has an astringent quality that helps bind the stools. Since it also has some ability to strengthen vital energy (Qi), it is an especially appropriate herb for this formula.

This is a very effective remedy that can also be used safely to treat diarrhea or excessive drooling in children, especially when they are underweight or malnourished. As always in the case of children, the dosage should be reduced in relation to the child's weight (see Clark's Rule in the dosage section of the Introduction).

Dosage: 12 pills, 3 times per day before meals

Manufacturer: Plum Flower; Sian Chinese Drug Pharmaceutical Works

Warnings and contraindications: This formula is inappropriate for acute diarrhea caused by bacteria, viruses, or parasites.

Shu Gan Wan

Pronunciation and translation: "shoo gahn wahn"— "soothe liver pill"

Indications: Digestive disorders which become worse under stress; abdominal distention and pain, nausea, belching, poor appetite, gas, and loose stools

Ingredients:

Bupleurum chinense root (Chai Hu)

Citrus aurantium fruit (Zhi Ke)

Glycyrrhiza uralensis root (Gan Cao)

Paeonia lactiflora root (Bai Shao)

Curcuma longa rhizome (Jiang Huang)

Aquilaria sinensis wood (Chen Xiang)

Corydalis yanhusuo rhizome (Yan Hu Suo)

Saussurea lappa root (Mu Xiang)

Magnolia officinalis bark (Hou Po)

Cyperus rotundus rhizome (Xiang Fu)

Paeonia suffruticosa root-bark (Mu Dan Pi)

Citrus medica fruit (Fo Shou)

Citrus reticulata peel (Chen Pi)

Citrus reticulata green peel (Qing Pi)

Amomum villosum seed (Sha Ren)

Amomum cardamomum fruit (Bai Dou Kou)

Santalum album wood (Tan Xiang)

Description: This is the standard formula for digestive difficulties due to an imbalance in the Liver. In traditional Chinese medicine, the Liver is responsible for the smooth flow of vital energy (Qi) in the body. When the Liver function becomes stagnant due to stress or environmental toxins, the effect is often felt in the digestive organs. Liver-related digestive problems will develop or get more severe under the influence of stress. There may also be a feeling of fullness and pain in the chest and abdominal area.

When this pattern occurs, it is important to use formulas that soothe the Liver in addition to herbs that resolve the digestive difficulties. This remedy addresses both areas. Bupleurum (Chai Hu), Turmeric (Jiang Huang), and Peony (Bai Shao) relax the Liver and eliminate the cause of the imbalance. Digestive strength is increased with two species of Cardamom (Bai Dou Kou and Sha Ren), while the distention and pain are eliminated with Qi-regulating herbs like Saussurea (Mu Xiang), Cyperus (Xiang Fu), and Corydalis (Yan Hu Suo). While this remedy will usually resolve the imbalance, it is important to reduce the sources of stress that can cause the problem. It is helpful to avoid alcohol and high-fat foods, and not to eat when hurried or upset.

Dosage: 8 pills, 3 times per day

Manufacturer: Lanzhou Foci

Warnings and contraindications: Do not use during pregnancy.

Wei Te Ling

Pronunciation and translation: "way tuh ling"—"stomach special effective"

Indications: Heartburn, excess stomach acid

Ingredients:

Sepia esculenta bone (Hai Piao Xiao)

Corydalis yanhusuo rhizome (Yan Hu Suo)

Apis mellifera honey (Feng Mi)

Description: Wei Te Ling is the herbal version of an over-the-counter antacid. It is a very simple formula, containing Cuttlefish bone (Hai Piao Xiao) as its chief ingredient. This astringent, calcium-rich substance neutralizes excess stomach acid and helps heal stomach ulcers. Corydalis (Yan Hu Suo) is a strong analgesic to relieve pain, and Honey (Feng Mi) is nourishing to the stomach lining. The combination of the three ingredients makes this a very useful remedy for heartburn, acid stomach, or simple ulcers.

Dosage: 4–6 pills, 3 times per day before meals, or as needed

Manufacturer: Tsingtao Medicine Works

Warnings and contraindications: It is best to avoid foods and habits that cause acid stomach, especially coffee, spicy foods, and over-eating.

Xiang Sha Liu Jun Wan; Aplotaxis Amomum Pills

Pronunciation and translation: "shahng shah loo juhn wahn"—"saussurea and cardamom six gentlemen pill"

Indications: Gastro-intestinal symptoms due to weak digestion, with symptoms of poor appetite, nausea, vomiting, belching, chronic diarrhea, and gurgling

Ingredients:

Codonopsis pilosula root (Dang Shen)

Atractylodes macrocephala rhizome (Bai Zhu)

Poria cocos fungus (Fu Ling)

Glycyrrhiza uralensis root (Gan Cao)

Pinellia ternata rhizome (Ban Xia)

Citrus reticulata peel (Chen Pi)

Saussurea lappa root (Mu Xiang)

Amomum villosum seed (Sha Ren)

Description: This is an augmented version of the basic tonic formula to strengthen digestion, which is known as Four Gentlemen Decoction. Its combination of Codonopsis, Atractylodes, Poria, and Licorice has a synergistic effect that enhances both the immune system and the body's ability to digest and assimilate food. When Pinellia and Citrus peel are added to further increase the digestive aspect, the formula is called Six Gentlemen Pills (Liu Jun Zi Wan). When this is further supplemented with Cardamom (Sha Ren) and Saussurea (Mu Xiang), the formula is called Xiang Sha Liu Jun Zi Wan. In this form, the remedy also has a strong ability to inhibit nausea in addition to its immune-stimulating and digestion-enhancing functions. For this reason, it is especially suitable for treating chemotherapy patients who are suffering from both nausea and depressed immunity. It is also quite useful for the symptoms of morning sickness and chronic gastritis.

Dosage: 12 pills, 3 times per day before meals

Manufacturer: Lanzhou Foci

Remedies for External Use: Plasters, Liniments, and Ointments

Ching Wan Hung; Jing Wan Hong
Pronunciation and translation: "ching wahn huhng"—"capital absolute red"
Indications: Burns of all kinds

Ingredients:
Chaenomeles lagenaria fruit (Mu Gua)
Sanguisorba officinalis root (Di Yu)
Boswellia carterii resin (Ru Xiang)
Lobelia chinensis plant (Ban Bian Lian)
Commiphora myrrh resin (Mo Yao)
Carthamus tinctorius flower (Hong Hua)
Angelica sinensis root (Dang Gui)
Dryobalanops aromatica crystal [Borneol camphor] (Bing Pian)

Description: Jing Wan Hong is one of the patent remedies that is absolutely essential in any home first aid or travel kit. In China, it is used for first, second, or third degree burns caused by hot water, steam, chemicals, radiation, or sunburn. The salve relieves pain very soon after it is applied, partly due to the analgesic action of Borneol camphor (Bing Pian). Damaged flesh is quickly regenerated, often with no scarring, since the formula also contains Myrrh (Mo Yao). Minor burns like sunburn can be healed remarkably fast, often in just a day or two.
Dosage: Apply externally as needed to cover the affected area.

Manufacturer: Tianjin Drug Manufactory
Warnings and contraindications: For external use only. This product can stain clothing.

Die Da Zhi Tong Gao; Plaster for Bruise and Analgesic

Pronunciation and translation: "dyeh dah juhr tuhng gow"—"contusion stop pain plaster"
Indications: Pain from sprains, traumatic injuries, or muscular tension

Ingredients:

Carthamus tinctorius flower (Hong Hua)
Commiphora myrrh resin (Mo Yao)
Daemonorops draco resin (Xue Jie)
Acacia catechu resin (Er Cha)
Eupolyphaga sinensis insect (Tu Bie Chong)
Dipsacus asper root (Xu Duan)
Drynaria fortunei rhizome (Gu Sui Bu)
Stegodon orientalis fossil (Long Gu)
Rheum palmatum rhizome (Da Huang)
Taraxacum mongolicum plant (Pu Gong Ying)
Mentha haplocalyx herb (Bo He)
Wintergreen oil (Dong Qing Yu)

Description: Herbal plasters are still commonly used in China today. They may seem like a throwback to pioneer days, but they actually work very well. The recommended brand is good, but there are others that are very similar, such as Hua Tuo Plasters and 701 Plasters. This particular brand, Plaster for Bruise and Analgesic, made by United Pharmaceutical Manufactory, comes in a larger size than the others, but it can be trimmed to size with scissors. The plaster consists of a self-adhering patch with an herbal concentrate mixed into the adhesive. A plastic backing is peeled away, and the plaster is applied to the sore area.

Herbal plasters relieve pain from sprains, strains, fractures, sports injuries, or premenstrual back soreness. In the case of spasmodic muscles, which frequently occur on the shoulders and upper back, the plaster can be applied directly to the tight area. If this is done before bed, the tightness will often be gone in the morning. It is best to apply the plaster to both sides in this case, since the tightness may travel to the other side if only the sore side is treated.

Plasters work by promoting the circulation of blood through the injured area, and it also has ingredients that reduce swelling, stop pain, and promote healing. Typically a plaster loses its potency after 24 hours and is then removed. To avoid irritation, it is best to let the skin air out for a few hours before putting on another plaster.

Dosage: As needed

Manufacturer: United Pharmaceutical Manufactory

Warnings and contraindications: Do not apply a plaster if the skin is broken. After 24 hours, remove the plaster and let the skin air out before applying more. Discontinue use if irritation develops. If the area to be treated has a lot of hair, it is best to use 701 brand plasters, since their adhesive is weaker.

Zheng Gu Shui

Pronunciation and translation: "juhng goo shway"— "setting bone liquid"

Indications: Traumatic injuries, bruises, fractures, sprains

Ingredients:

Panax pseudoginseng root, foliage, and flower (Tian Qi)

Angelica dahurica root (Bai Zhi)

Croton crassifolium root (Ji Gu Xiang)

Mentha haplocalyx crystal (Bo He Nao)

Cinnamomum camphora crystal (Zhang Nao)

Tiglii seed (Wu Ma Xun Cheng)

Moghania phillipinensis root (Qian Jin Ba)

Inula cappa (Da Li Wang)

Description: As its name suggests, Zheng Gu Shui ("setting bone liquid") is especially suitable for promoting healing in fractured or bruised bones. In China, it is applied to the area before the bone is set in the hospital. After the bone is set, the area of the fracture is covered with cotton soaked in the liniment. The procedure is repeated twice daily until healing occurs. While this may not be practical when a plaster cast is used, it can be done when there is a removable cast or when a cast is not needed. It can also be used for sore feet, sprains, or sports injuries if the skin is not broken.

Dosage: Apply externally as needed.

Manufacturer: Tulin Drug Manufactory

Warnings and contraindications: For external use only. Wash hands thoroughly after applying. Stains clothing. Do not use on open wounds. Discontinue use immediately if a skin reaction develops. Keep tightly closed and out of reach of children. This liquid is flammable; keep away from open flame. Do not expose the treated skin to full sun when the liniment is applied.

Remedies for the Immune System and Overall Wellness (Tonics)

Central Qi Pills; Bu Zhong Yi Qi Wan

Pronunciation and translation: "boo juhng yee chee wahn"—"tonify the middle, strengthen Qi pills"

Indications: Deficiency of Qi (vital energy), weak digestion, prolapsed organs

Ingredients:

Astragalus membranaceus root (Huang Qi)

Codonopsis pilosula root (Dang Shen)

Atractylodes macrocephala rhizome (Bai Zhu)

Glycyrrhiza uralensis root (Gan Cao)

Angelica sinensis root (Dang Gui)

Citrus reticulata peel (Chen Pi)

Cimicifuga foetida rhizome (Sheng Ma)

Bupleurum chinense root (Chai Hu)

Zingiberis officinalis fresh rhizome (Sheng Jiang)

Ziziphus jujuba fruit (Da Zao)

Description: Bu Zhong Yi Qi Wan is the standard formula for organs that are prolapsed (sagging) due to a deficiency of Qi (vital energy). In addition to prolapse, other symptoms could include fatigue, poor appetite, loose stools, and a tendency to feel cold. This formula is an energetic combination of herbs that strengthen the Qi along with herbs that exert an uplifting action. In Chinese medicine, herbs are sometimes classified according to their directional activity. Two of the herbs in this formula, Bupleurum and Cimicifuga, are often selected for their ability to direct a formula upward, although they also have other therapeutic actions.

There is some modern research to support the use of this classical formula. In one clinical trial, 103 people with gastroptosis (prolapse of the Stomach) were treated with a decoction of this formula. All but two of the people in the trial experienced either full recovery or some improvement. In another study, twenty-three women with prolapsed uterus took the decoction version of this formula for two weeks. Out of the twenty-one women who finished the treatment, sixteen experienced full recovery, two improved, and only three showed no improvement.

Bu Zhong Yi Qi Wan is also commonly used to strengthen women who experience miscarriages due to Qi deficiency.

Dosage: 8 pills, 3 times per day

Manufacturer: Lanzhou Foci

Warnings and contraindications: For the above conditions, seek the help of a qualified health care practitioner before using this remedy.

Ginseng Royal Jelly Vials; Renshen Feng Wang Jiang

Pronunciation and translation: "ren shen fuhng wahng jyahng"—"ginseng and royal jelly syrup"

Indications: Fatigue, poor appetite, feeling cold and weak

Ingredients:
Panax ginseng root (Ren Shen)
Royal jelly (Feng Wang)

Description: Ginseng is without a doubt the most well known of all Chinese herbs. What other herb from Asia can be commonly found at checkout lines of convenience stores and gas stations? This product isn't nearly as strong as an extract of Ginseng derived by boiling a root for an hour; powdered extracts of the root are also stronger. On the other hand, these little vials are very convenient, and they can provide a much-needed boost of energy during strenuous activity. Be sure to use a reputable brand that actually contains Ginseng and is free of caffeine or other adulterants.

It is important to be aware of the difference between the various types of Ginseng. There are three true species: Panax ginseng, Panax quinquifolium, and Panax notoginseng. Panax notoginseng is used mostly for injuries, and it is the main ingredient in Yunnan Pai Yao (see p. 64). Panax quinquifolium is commonly known as American Ginseng. Its main distinction is that it has a cooling effect on the body. This makes it more appropriate for use in hot weather or for people with a red face, rapid pulse, irritability, and a tendency to overheat easily. A person like this will experience adverse effects from Asian Ginseng (Panax ginseng), which is very warming. Some possible side effects could be headache, stiff neck, irritability, skin rash, or a feverish feeling. Panax ginseng is the herb of choice for people who tend to look pale and feel cold, and it is indicated for low immunity, fatigue, and a host of other ailments. When it is combined with Royal jelly, as in this product, its effects are enhanced.

Ginseng has been investigated extensively, especially by the Russians and the Chinese. It is considered to be an adaptogen, meaning it helps an organism to adapt to severe stresses in the environment. Some of Ginseng's therapeutic effects include the following:

1. Reduces fatigue
2 Reduces the toxicity of certain chemicals
3. Stimulates the pituitary and adrenal cortex
4. Reduces blood sugar levels and is synergistic with insulin
5. Regulates cholesterol levels
6. Increases absorption of nutrients in the digestive system
7. Increases the body's immune response
8. Normalizes blood count
9. Stimulates production of immune globulins

After scanning this partial list of Ginseng's actions, it is easy to see why it has such an enduring reputation as a tonic for multiple purposes. When used wisely and appropriately, it can have a powerful ability to support us in our toxic and stressful modern lives.

Dosage: 1–2 vials per day.

Manufacturer: Harbin 3rd Pharmaceutical Manufactory

Warnings and contraindications: Panax ginseng is very warming. It is not appropriate for a person who has *heat* signs, such as a red face, irritability, rapid pulse, restlessness, and a tendency to feel warm. Discontinue use if any of the above symptoms, or headache or stiff neck develop after taking Ginseng.

Imperial Astragali Extract; Bei Qi Jing

Pronunciation and translation: "bay chee jing"—"essence of northern astragalus"

Indications: Fatigue, weak immunity

Ingredients:

Astragalus membranaceus root (Huang Qi)

Honey (Feng Mi)

Description: The medicinal use of Astragalus root is one of the great contributions of Chinese herbal medicine. For thousands of years, it has been used to strengthen the Wei Qi ("way chee"), which is the ancients' way of describing the immune system. From a scientific perspective, Astragalus increases the production of antibodies and macrophages and improves resistance to stress. These are all important components of the body's immune response. The root slices, which look like tongue depressors, are often boiled into soup broth to be used as a daily wellness tonic. Other uses for this versatile herb include strengthening digestion, reducing edema, and regenerating flesh that is lost by injury or surgery. When combined with Ligustrum fruit (Nu Zhen Zi), it can also normalize the blood count after chemotherapy.

While this patent medicine is a convenient way to use Astragalus, the effect is much stronger when the sliced roots are boiled into a decoction. It is also available in other forms, such as dehydrated crystals.

Dosage: 1–2 vials per day

Manufacturer: Plum Flower

Warnings and contraindications: While Astragalus can help prevent colds or infections, it is not recommended if they have already occurred. This is because Astragalus shuts down the pores, which prevents the body from expelling a pathogen. The Chinese call this "trapping the burglar," meaning it is counterproductive to lock all the doors if a burglar is already in the house. Once the pathogen has been expelled with remedies like Gan Mao Ling (see p. 76) or Yin Qiao Jie Du Pian (see p. 81), it is appropriate to use Astragalus to protect the body from future infections.

Ling Zhi Beverage

Pronunciation and translation: "ling juhr"
Indications: Frequent colds, chronic bronchitis, high cholesterol, stress

Ingredients:

Ganoderma lucidum fungus (Ling Zhi)

Description: Ganoderma (Ling Zhi), commonly known as Reishi, its Japanese name, is a beautiful, glossy black or red fungus that grows on trees in the wild. Prior to the 1970s, when researchers learned to cultivate it, Reishi was exceptionally rare and expensive. For example, in a grove of two hundred thousand plum trees, only seven wild Reishi mushrooms were found. It doesn't usually appear in the traditional herbal formulas, because it was formerly reserved for use by the emperor. Now that it can be grown in the laboratory from spores, it is widely available at a reasonable price. This particular product is an extract of the fungus, and it can be dissolved in water. A much stronger concentration can be obtained by boiling the fungus in water for an hour. Dehydrated crystals and liquid extracts are also available at retail herb and supplement stores.

Reishi has a quality that is unique among herbs that build vital energy (Qi): it is actually able to sedate and tranquilize a person while it energizes. This makes it especially appropriate for individuals who are weak and depleted but also nervous and irritable. This precious fungus has some important cardiovascular actions as well. It improves circulation to the coronary artery and heart muscles, and it decreases oxygen consumption by the heart. It also lowers blood pressure and cholesterol levels, making it exceptionally useful in maintaining cardiovascular health. Reishi is commonly included in formulas to stimulate the immune system, because it enhances immunity, increases white blood cell counts, and has antibacterial activity. It is also an antitussive and expectorant, making it an effective treatment for chronic bronchitis. Like Ginseng, it is considered a true herbal panacea.

Dosage: 1 cube, dissolved in water

Manufacturer: Guangxi Medicines and Health Products

Liu Wei Di Huang Wan; Rehmannia Six Teapills; Six Flavor Tea

Pronunciation and translation: "loo way dee hwahng wahn"—"six ingredient rehmannia pills"

Indications: Thirst, irritability, night sweats, insomnia, weak lower back and knees

Ingredients:

Rehmannia glutinosa prepared root (Shu Di Huang)

Dioscorea opposita root (Shan Yao)

Cornus officinalis fruit (Shan Zhu Yu)

Poria cocos fungus (Fu Ling)

Alisma plantago-aquatica rhizome (Ze Xie)

Paeonia suffruticosa root-bark (Mu Dan Pi)

Description: This is the classical base formula for all conditions of Yin deficiency, especially of the Liver and Kidneys. The Yin aspect of an organ refers to its structure and substance, while the Yang aspect refers to its functions and activities. Yin is cooling and moist; Yang is warming and dry. The Yin aspect of the body works as a lubricant, calming and enriching the organs. It can become deficient due to a variety of factors, such as over-work, lack of sufficient rest or fluid intake, stress, an overly dry environment, or excessive sexual activity. When Yin is deficient, there can be chronic *dryness* and inflammation. This can be compared to running a car that is low on oil or water. The lack of lubrication or coolant will cause the engine to run hotter than normal; continued operation under these conditions can lead to long-term damage.

Symptoms of Liver and Kidney Yin deficiency include a warm sensation in the sternum, palms, and soles of the feet; red cheeks; night sweats; a feeling of heat and irritability in the afternoon and evening; sore and weak low back and knees; tinnitus (ringing in the ears); chronic dry mouth and thirst. The tongue will often be reddish with little or no coating, and the pulse typically feels thin and rapid. By focusing on nourishing the Yin and clearing the *heat* caused by the deficiency, this formula subtly and elegantly treats a wide range of seemingly unrelated symptoms. It contains three ingredients that nourish the Yin and three that clear *heat*.

The chief tonifying herb in the formula is Rehmannia glutinosa (Shu Di Huang). In its raw state, it has a cold energy and nourishes the Yin, making it useful in the treatment of high fevers and in alleviating thirst due to diabetes. In its prepared form, it is treated with wine, making it more nourishing to the Blood. In this form, it is used to treat anemia and menstrual difficulties and as an overall tonic to the Kidneys and adrenals.

Another important ingredient is Dioscorea (Shan Yao), a tonic to the Lungs, Stomach, and Kidneys. It also stimulates the immune system to produce interferon, a substance that suppresses viruses without disturbing normal body functions.

The third tonic herb is Cornus officinalis (Shan Zhu Yu), an astringent herb with a variety of actions: it is antiallergic, diuretic, anti-hypertensive, antitumor, antibacterial, and anti-fungal; and it increases the production of white blood cells. Being astringent, it energetically prevents further depletion of Yin through the excessive loss of semen, perspiration, urine, or uterine blood. It acts to consolidate the effect of the other tonifying herbs.

Alisma plantago (Ze Xie) is an important diuretic herb that grows wild in North America. It has a strong diuretic action, and it lowers blood pressure for prolonged periods of time. In addition to antibacterial qualities, it is an important herb for lowering blood sugar and cholesterol, another reason this formula is effective in treating diabetes. Poria cocos (Fu Ling) is another diuretic herb that also has a calming effect on the body. It is one of the important herbs for stimulating deep immunity; it induces interferon production and contains polysaccharides that stimulate macrophages to track down and destroy cells that are foreign to the body. The final herb in the formula is Mouton root bark (Mu Dan Pi), an aromatic agent that is cooling to the body on a number of different levels. It kills staphylococcus bacteria, lowers blood pressure, and decreases body temperature.

This is a highly sophisticated formula that is useful in a wide variety of conditions that manifest with the designated symptoms. There are numerous modifications to this base formula, depending on the particular focus. Some of the disorders that can be treated with Liu Wei Di Huang Wan are: diabetes, tuberculosis, hyperthyroidism, nephritis, hypertension, chronic urinary tract infection, and various degenerative diseases of the eye. In some cases, such as tuberculosis, Western pharmaceuticals would be taken along with the herbs. Obviously, many of these are serious conditions that should not be self-treated. As with most of the remedies in this book, it is essential to be under the care of a qualified physician while using these herbs. Many variations of this formula are available for specific ailments; Zhi Bai Di Huang Wa (see p. 96) and Ming Mu Di Huang Wan, discussed below, are also discussed in this book.

Dosage: 8–10 pills, 3 times per day

Manufacturer: Lanzhou Foci

Warnings and contraindications: Rehmannia can be difficult to digest, so this formula should be discontinued if excessive loose stools become a problem.

Ming Mu Di Huang Wan

Pronunciation and translation: "ming moo dee hwahng wahn"—"brighten eyes rehmannia pills"

Indications: Dry eyes, blurry vision, poor eyesight

Ingredients:

Rehmannia glutinosa prepared root (Shu Di Huang)

Dioscorea opposita root (Shan Yao)

Cornus officinalis fruit (Shan Zhu Yu)

Poria cocos fungus (Fu Ling)

Alisma plantago-aquatica rhizome (Ze Xie)

Paeonia suffruticosa root-bark (Mu Dan Pi)

Lycium chinensis fruit (Gou Qi Zi)

Haliotis diversicolor shell (Shi Jue Ming)

Tribulus terrestris fruit (Bai Ji Li)

Description: Ming Mu Di Huang Wan is a variation of the previous formula, Liu Wei Di Huang Wan. This formula contains ingredients that focus on eye problems caused by the underlying problem of Yin deficiency, such as blurry vision, dry eyes, night blindness, and excessive tears. There may also be the general signs of Yin deficiency: dry mouth and throat, night sweats, and a sensation of heat in the palms and soles of the feet.

One of the additional herbs, Lycium fruit (Gou Qi Zi), is actually quite good to eat. It looks and tastes like raisins. These fruits are nourishing to the Liver Yin, which is the basis for healthy eyes. From a Western pharmacological perspective, Lycium fruit is hepato-protective, helping the liver eliminate toxic substances. In Chinese herbalism, it is specifically used to "brighten the eyes." The other two additions to the base formula are Abalone shell (Shi Jue Ming) and Tribulus fruit (Bai Ji Li); these are both specific for eye problems caused by *heat* in the Liver, making them appropriate for this remedy.

It is important to have an accurate diagnosis before using this formula. Similar eye problems can be due to a different heat pattern, and they require completely different herbs. For example, conjunctivitis due to Liver fire would require the formula Long Dan Xie Gan Wan (see p. 87), while red eyes due to Yin deficiency would be treated with this formula. This is another example of why a diagnosis from an acupuncturist is important before attempting to use this book for self-treatment.

Dosage: 10 pills, 3 times per day

Manufacturer: Lanzhou Foci

Warnings and contraindications: Not for red or swollen eyes due to conjunctivitis. Rehmannia can be difficult to digest, so this formula should be discontinued if excessive loose stools become a problem.

Shen Qi Da Bu Wan

Pronunciation and translation: "shen chee dah boo wahn"—"codonopsis astragalus great tonifying pill"

Indications: Weak immunity, fatigue, lack of appetite

Ingredients:

Codonopsis pilosula root (Dang Shen)

Astragalus membranaceus root (Huang Qi)

Description: This is a very simple formula to revive the vital energy (Qi), especially after a long illness, chemotherapy, or blood loss. This is also a good remedy to enhance the immune system (Wei Qi). The immune-stimulating properties of Astragalus are described in detail under Imperial Astragali Extract (see p. 49). When combined with Codonopsis pilosula (Dang Shen), these effects are enhanced. Codonopsis is often used as a substitute for Ginseng, since it is less warming and less expensive. It is an excellent tonic that increases red and white blood cell counts, making it very effective along with Astragalus in recovering from chemotherapy or radiation.

Both Astragalus and Codonopsis have a pleasant, mild, sweet taste. The roots are often boiled and used in soup stocks for a Chinese version of preventive medicine. They are fairly easy to grow, and seeds are available from a number of suppliers. If you live in an area with gophers, be sure to protect your plant beds with wire cages. Otherwise, after the roots get nice and juicy, they will suddenly disappear and you'll have a lot of gophers with strong immune systems!

Dosage: 8–10 pills, 3 times per day

Manufacturer: Lanzhou Foci

Remedies for Men

Kai Kit Wan

Pronunciation and translation: "keye kit wahn"—"dispel knot pills"

Indications: Benign swelling of the prostate gland

Ingredients:

Vaccaria segetalis seed (Wang Bu Liu Xing)

Patrinia scabiosaefolia plant (Bai Jiang Cao)

Paeonia lactiflora root (Bai Shao)

Astragalus membranaceus root (Huang Qi)

Paeonia suffruticosa root-bark (Mu Dan Pi)

Akebia trifoliata stem (Mu Tong)

Glycyrrhiza uralensis root (Gan Cao)

Saussurea lappa root (Mu Xiang)

Corydalis yanhusuo rhizome (Yan Hu Suo)

Description: Benign prostatic hypertrophy (non-cancerous swelling of the prostate gland) is very common in men over fifty years of age. Typical symptoms are difficulty in urination, frequent urination, dripping of urine, and interruption of urine flow. All of these symptoms are caused by the swelling of the prostate gland, which surrounds the urethra. Energetically, the swelling can be considered a stagnation of Qi and Blood, with a likely accumulation of *heat* and *dampness*. For this reason, treatment includes herbs that promote circulation and reduce *dampness* and stagnation. The chief herb in this formula is Vaccaria seed (Wang Bu Liu Xing), which has an affinity for promoting circulation in the sexual organs. Another important ingredient is Patrinia (Bai Jiang

Cao), which clears stagnation and *dampness*. It also has an affinity for the male reproductive organs, being used with Vaccaria for testicular swelling due to mumps. Combined with the other herbs in the formula, which strengthen vital energy, promote circulation, and relieve pain, this remedy can help reduce the swelling. It is recommended to include Saw palmetto berries (Serenoa repens) in the treatment protocol, since they are a well-researched and effective treatment for this condition. Saw palmetto is available in most health food or supplement stores.

Dosage: 2–3 pills, 3 times per day

Manufacturer: Plum Flower

Warnings and contraindications: Men over age fifty should be screened for prostate cancer before attempting self-treatment for prostate problems.

Remedies for the Musculoskeletal System

Jin Gu Die Shang Wan
Pronunciation and translation: "jin goo dyeh shahng wahn"—"muscles and bones injury pill"
Indications: Traumatic injuries, bruises, sprains, and swelling

Ingredients:
Panax notoginseng root (Tian Qi)
Paeonia rubra root (Chi Shao)
Prunus persica seed (Tao Ren)
Boswellia carterii resin (Ru Xiang)
Commiphora myrrha resin (Mo Yao)
Curcuma longa rhizome (Jiang Huang)
Paeonia suffruticosa root-bark (Mu Dan Pi)
Caesalpinia sappan wood (Su Mu)
Drynaria fortunei rhizome (Gu Sui Bu)
Sparganium stoloniferum rhizome (San Leng)
Daeomonorops draco resin (Xue Jie)
Artemisia anomala plant (Liu Ji Nu)
Angelica sinensis root (Dang Gui)
Dipsacus japonicus root (Xu Duan)
Siler divaricata root (Fang Feng)
Cucumis seed (Tian Gua Zi)
Citrus aurantium fruit (Zhi Ke)
Glycyrrhiza uralensis root (Gan Cao)
Platycodon grandiflorum root (Jie Geng)
Akebia trifoliata stem (Mu Tong)
Pyritum mineral (Zi Ran Tong)
Eupolyphaga sinensis insect (Tu Bie Chong)

Description: Jin Gu Die Shang Wan is used to treat traumatic injuries. It is a combination of a large number of herbs that stimulate blood circulation, reduce swelling, stop pain, and promote healing. When combined with one of the liniments or plasters for external application, it can bring relief very quickly. Unlike Western practitioners, who use ice for traumatic injury, Chinese herbalists believe that the stagnation of Qi and Blood should be treated with warming herbs that increase circulation to the area. While ice is very helpful in reducing swelling in the first few hours after an injury, it can actually hinder the healing process after the swelling is stabilized. When the initial swelling is under control, improved circulation to the injured area helps to carry away waste materials and bring nutrients to repair the damage.

Dosage: 8 pills, 3 times per day

Manufacturer: Plum Flower

Warnings and contraindications: Not to be used during pregnancy. Plum Flower brand is recommended and is free of heavy metals. An alternative brand tested positive for low levels of heavy metals.

Du Huo Jisheng Wan

Pronunciation and translation: "doo hwaw jee shuhng wahn"—"angelica loranthus pills"

Indications: Chronic pain and stiffness in the low back and knees; arthritis

Ingredients:

Angelica pubescens root (Du Huo)

Gentiana macrophylla root (Qin Jiao)

Siler divaricata root (Fang Feng)

Asarum sieboldi plant (Xi Xin)

Eucommia ulmoidis bark (Du Zhong)

Achyranthes bidentata root (Niu Xi)

Loranthus parasiticus stem and branch (Sang Ji Sheng)

Angelica sinensis root (Dang Gui)

Ligusticum wallichii root (Chuan Xiong)

Rehmannia glutinosa prepared root (Shu Di Huang)

Paeonia lactiflora root (Bai Shao)

Codonopsis pilosula root (Dang Shen)

Poria cocos fungus (Fu Ling)

Glycyrrhiza uralensis root (Gan Cao)

Description: This is an excellent remedy for elderly people, since it is a well-formulated combination of herbs that tonify and strengthen the body along with herbs that improve circulation and reduce pain. It is especially helpful for pain in the low back and knees. This is due to the Achyranthes (Niu Xi), which literally means "cow's knee," and Angelica pubescens (Du Huo), an effective analgesic for pain in the lower part of the body. The formula also contains the basic combination to strengthen Qi and Blood, along with herbs that build the Yang of the Kidneys. Since pain in the low back and knees is a sign of Kidney weakness, this remedy addresses the underlying cause of the pain in addition to treating the symptoms. It is most appropriate for pain that becomes worse in cold and damp weather.

Dosage: 8 pills, 3 times per day

Manufacturer: Plum Flower

Warnings and contraindications: Contraindicated for use during pregnancy. Not to be used for inflamed joints that feel hot. Plum Flower brand contains no acetaminophen, which has been detected in another brand.

Yan Hu Suo Pian
Pronunciation and translation: "yahn hoo swaw pyen"—
"corydalis tablets"
Indications: Headache, menstrual pain

Ingredients:
Corydalis yanhusuo tuber (Yan Hu Suo)
Angelica dahurica root (Bai Zhi)

Description: Corydalis rhizome (Yan Hu Suo) is one of the
best pain-relieving herbs in Chinese medicine. The alcohol
and acetic acid extracts are the strongest, being 40 percent as
effective as morphine. It is especially useful in treating menstrual pain, but it can also be used for chest or abdominal
pain or pain due to injuries or hernia. When combined with
Angelica dahurica (Bai Zhi), as in this formula, it can also
treat headache due to the common cold or sinus congestion.
Dosage: 4 pills, 3 times per day
Manufacturer: Plum Flower
Warnings and contraindications:

1. Not to be used during pregnancy.

2. Do not confuse this product with Yan Hu Su Zhi Tong
   Pian, which has similar uses but contains a pharmaceutical. The word Su in the name refers to an individual
   chemical constituent isolated from an herb, in this case
   tetrahydropalmatine, a strong analgesic drug. There is
   also a 100 percent herbal version known as Yan Hu Suo
   Zhi Tong Pian.

3. This remedy only provides symptomatic relief. It is important to treat the underlying cause, especially of chest and abdominal pain, since these can be symptoms of serious disease.

Yunnan Pai Yao

Pronunciation and translation: "yuhnahn peye yow"— "white medicine from Yunnan"

Indications: Bleeding of any kind, bruises or sports injuries, menstrual pain

Ingredients:

Panax notoginseng root (Tian Qi)
The medicine is white. A red emergency pill is included to be used in case of shock. Ingredients in the red emergency pill are a family secret.

Description: Yunnan Pai Yao is one of the essential patent medicines for the home or traveling first aid kit. Its ability to stop pain, swelling, and bleeding is legendary. The main ingredient, Panax notoginseng (Tian Qi), has a powerful ability to shorten bleeding time. In fact, during the war in Vietnam, Vietcong guerrillas were often found with a vial of this medicine around their neck, to be used in case of gunshot wounds. This formula has been a family secret for generations, and it is therefore one of the few remedies that still meets the criteria for the Chinese version of "patent medicine." While the formula itself contains mostly Tian Qi Ginseng, very little is known about the composition of the little "red emergency pill," which is taken when extensive bleeding is leading to shock.

When used for bruises and injuries, this remedy can greatly speed up the healing process. It is well known for resolving serious bruising and swelling in a matter of days. It is also used by midwives to stop any excessive bleeding after delivery. Yunnan Pai Yao is also available in powder form and as a liquid for external application.

Dosage: 2 capsules, 3 or 4 times per day

Manufacturer: Yunnan Paiyao Factory

Warnings and contraindications: Not to be used during pregnancy. Serious injuries should always be inspected by a physician to detect possible fractures or internal bleeding.

Remedies for the Nervous System

An Mien Pian
Pronunciation and translation: "ahn myehn pyen"—
"peaceful sleep tablets"
Indications: Insomnia, anxiety

Ingredients:
Zizyphus spinosa seed (Suan Zao Ren)
Polygala tenuifolia root (Yuan Zhi)
Poria cocos fungus (Fu Ling)
Gardenia jasminoidis fruit (Zhi Zi)
Fermentata medicinalis mass (Shen Qu)
Glycyrrhiza uralensis root (Gan Cao)

Description: An Mien Pian is a mild sedative that can be used safely by frail or elderly people. It is useful for anxiety, insomnia, excessive dreaming, or poor memory, all signs of a deficiency of the Yin cooling system of the Heart. The chief ingredients are Zizyphus seed (Suan Zao Ren) and Polygala root (Yuan Zhi), both of which are considered to "nourish the Heart and calm the spirit." Poria fungus (Fu Ling) and Fermented mass (Shen Qu) are included to help indigestion, which can cause insomnia. Gardenia fruit (Zhi Zi) helps to eliminate internal *heat*, which can cause restlessness. This formula can be taken for a long period of time due to its mild nature.
Dosage: 4 tablets, 3 times per day
Manufacturer: Plum Flower

Emperor's Tea; Tian Wang Bu Xin Dan

Pronunciation and translation: "tyahn wahng boo shin dahn"—"emperor of heaven's pill to tonify the heart"

Indications: Insomnia, palpitations, anxiety, night sweats

Ingredients:

Rehmannia glutinosa root (Sheng Di Huang)

Angelica sinensis root (Dang Gui)

Schisandra chinensis fruit (Wu Wei Zi)

Zizyphus spinosa seed (Suan Zao Ren)

Biota orientalis seed (Bai Zi Ren)

Asparagus cochinchinensis tuber (Tian Men Dong)

Ophiopogon japonicus tuber (Mai Men Dong)

Scrophularia ningpoensis root (Xuan Shen)

Salvia miltiorrhiza root (Dan Shen)

Codonopsis pilosula root (Dang Shen)

Poria cocos fungus (Fu Ling)

Platycodon grandiflorum root (Jie Geng)

Polygala tenuifolia root (Yuan Zhi)

Description: Emperor's Tea is the standard treatment for the pattern known as Heart Yin deficiency. This pattern may relate to the actual heart organ, but in Chinese diagnosis it is important to remember that an energetic description like Heart Yin may not always involve the heart organ itself. The Yin of the Heart gets depleted from lack of sleep, overwork, stress, or poor diet. This causes the Heart to become overheated, with symptoms such as palpitations, insomnia, restlessness, anxiety, intense dreams, and possibly thirst and night sweats. The formula goes to the root of the problem by including substances that nourish the Heart Yin and calm the spirit.

The chief ingredient in the remedy is Rehmannia root (Sheng Di Huang), which nourishes the Yin and helps clear some of the *heat* resulting from the lack of lubrication. It is combined with Scrophularia root (Xuan Shen) and Asparagus root (Tian Men Dong) to enhance the cooling effect. Salvia (Dan Shen) is incorporated to increase circulation to the coronary artery and allow the heart to work with a lower oxygen requirement. When combined with Schisandra berries (Wu Wei Zi), the palpitations can be relieved. To relieve the insomnia, nourishing herbs are used that also have a calming effect: Biota seed (Bai Zi Ren), Zizyphus seed (Suan Zao Ren), and Polygala root (Yuan Zhi). In order to replenish the exhausted reserves of Qi and Blood, the formula also includes Codonopsis root (Dang Shen) and Angelica sinensis root (Dang Gui).

If the symptoms support a diagnosis of Heart Yin deficiency, this remedy can be useful in treating mouth ulcers, hyperthyroidism, insomnia, hypertension, or chronic fatigue. A visit to a qualified acupuncturist or Chinese herbalist can confirm the diagnosis.

Dosage: 8 pills, 3 times per day
The formula should be taken for a few months to have a long-lasting effect.

Manufacturer: Lanzhou Foci

Warnings and contraindications: As with all formulas containing large amounts of Rehmannia, discontinue use if loose stools become a problem.

Gui Pi Wan; Angelica Longan Tea

Pronunciation and translation: "gway pee wahn"—"bring back the spleen pills"

Indications: Fatigue, palpitations, poor memory, insomnia

Ingredients:

Codonopsis pilosula root (Dang Shen)
Poria cocos fungus (Fu Shen)
Zizyphus spinosa seed (Suan Zao Ren)
Polygala tenuifolia root (Yuan Zhi)
Angelica sinensis root (Dang Gui)
Saussurea lappa root (Mu Xiang)
Atractylodes macrocephala rhizome (Bai Zhu)
Glycyrrhiza uralensis root (Gan Cao)
Euphoria longan fruit (Long Yan Rou)
Astragalus membranaceus root (Huang Qi)

Description: Gui Pi Wan is one of the classical ancient formulas that is available as a patent medicine. It is indicated for patterns that involve both the nervous system (Heart) and digestive system (Spleen). It is especially useful for "student's syndrome," where both of these organ systems have become depleted due to excessive studying and lack of exercise. The Heart deficiency symptoms are palpitations, insomnia, poor memory, and intense dreams; the Spleen deficiency symptoms could include fatigue, low appetite, pale face, and excessive menstrual bleeding with light-colored blood.

Since the formula treats deficiency in two different organ systems, the ingredients reflect this duality. Ingredients that tonify the Spleen include Codonopsis (Dang Shen), Poria (Fu Shen), Saussurea (Mu Xiang), Atractylodes (Bai Zhu), Licorice (Gan Cao), and Astragalus (Huang Qi). Herbs that deal with the Heart symptoms are Zizyphus (Suan Zao Ren), Polygala (Yuan Zhi), Angelica (Dang Gui), and Longan (Long Yan Rou).

Although the Heart and Spleen symptoms may seem unrelated, there is a strong connection between them. When the digestive energy (Spleen Qi) is strong, more nutrients are assimilated from food. This enables the body to produce more Blood, which in turn nourishes the Heart. Conversely, when the Heart Blood is sufficient, the digestive organs receive the nutrients that are needed for optimal function. This symbiotic relationship is nicely explained in the ancient Chinese saying, "Blood is the mother of Qi, and Qi is the leader of Blood." This refers to the fact that without Blood, there is no fundamental nutritional basis for Qi; without Qi, there would be no ability to form or circulate Blood, and it would fail to stay within the vessels. This formula is a practical application of this ancient principle.

Dosage: 8 pills, 3 times per day

Manufacturer: Lanzhou Foci

Remedies for the Respiratory System

Bi Yan Pian

Pronunciation and translation: "bee yahn pyen"—"nose inflammation tablets"

Indications: Nasal congestion, allergies, rhinitis, sinusitis

Ingredients:

Xanthium sibiricum fruit (Cang Er Zi)
Magnolia liliflora flower (Xin Yi Hua)
Glycyrrhiza uralensis root (Gan Cao)
Phellodendron amurense bark (Huang Bai)
Platycodon grandiflorum root (Jie Geng)
Schisandra chinensis fruit (Wu Wei Zi)
Forsythia suspensa fruit (Lian Qiao)
Angelica dahurica root (Bai Zhi)
Anemarrhena asphodeloides rhizome (Zhi Mu)
Chrysanthemum indica flower (Ye Ju Hua)
Siler divaricata root (Fang Feng)
Schizonepeta tenuifolia herb (Jing Jie)

Description: Bi Yan Pian is a widely used and popular remedy for problems related to the nasal passages or sinuses. It can be used in both acute and chronic conditions whenever there is congestion, runny nose, or excessive mucus in these areas. It can effectively treat allergies to pollen, animal dander, mold, or any substance that causes nasal congestion and sneezing. The ingredients that make this such a useful remedy for nasal congestion are Xanthium fruit (Cang Er Zi), Magnolia flower (Xin Yi Hua), and Angelica dahurica root

(Bai Zhi). The formula also contains Siler root (Fang Feng) and Schizonepeta flower (Jing Jie), which help the immune system fight off colds (external *wind*). There are also cooling ingredients, including Phellodendron bark (Huang Bai), Forsythia fruit (Lian Qiao), Anemarrhena rhizome (Zhi Mu), and Wild Chrysanthemum flower (Ye Ju Hua), that help to prevent infection. However, if a sinus infection has already developed, Bi Yan Pian should be supplemented with a formula that will help fight the infection, such as Chuan Xin Lian. When the congestion is due to the common cold, it can be taken along with Gan Mao Ling (see p. 76) or Yin Qiao Jie Du Pian (see p. 81). Many people have found this remedy to be as effective as over-the-counter decongestants with none of the uncomfortable side effects like drowsiness or over-stimulation.

Dosage: 4 pills, 3 times per day

Manufacturer: Plum Flower

Warnings and contraindications: It is preferable to use a brand such as Plum Flower, that does not contain acetaminophen or artificial coloring. Do not exceed the recommended dosage. If a sinus infection does not resolve or symptoms get worse, seek medical attention immediately. If the nasal passages, mouth, or throat get excessively dry when using this formula, decrease the dosage or discontinue its use.

Chuan Xin Lian Antiphlogistic Tablets

Pronunciation and translation: "chwahn shin lyahn"— "andrographis anti-inflammatory tablets"

Indications: Inflammation due to excess *heat*, swollen glands, severe sore throat, viral and bacterial infections

Ingredients:

Andrographis paniculata herb (Chuan Xin Lian)

Taraxacum mongolicum plant (Pu Gong Ying)

Isatis tinctoria root (Ban Lan Gen)

Description: This remedy clears *heat* and inflammation from all areas of the body. It can be used for severe sore throat, coughs with yellow phlegm, urinary tract infections, or dysentery. The formula gets its name from the chief ingredient, Andrographis paniculata herb (Chuan Xin Lian). This extremely bitter herb has powerful antibacterial and antiviral properties. Clinical studies have shown it to inhibit the growth of the bacteria that cause streptococcal and staphylococcal infections, pneumonia, and dysentery. It also increases phagocytosis, the ability of white blood cells to destroy bacteria. In China, it is commonly used to treat acute infections of the respiratory, digestive, and urinary tracts.

Another ingredient that has strong antibacterial activity is the common Dandelion, Taraxacum mongolicum (Pu Gong Ying). It inhibits the same bacteria as Andrographis, as well as those that cause meningitis and diphtheria. It is strange that in our culture, we spray deadly herbicides to kill a plant with such powerful healing properties! Recent studies have also shown a higher rate of cancer in children who play in areas that have been treated with these toxic chemicals. A change in our perception of wild plants, as well as our response to them, seems to be in order. While technology has brought many miracles, we still have a lot to learn from the ancient cultures.

The third ingredient in this patent medicine is Isatis tinctoria root (Ban Lan Gen). Like the other herbs, it has a cooling, antibacterial effect on infections and inflammation.

Isatis is also antiviral; clinical studies have proved it to be highly effective in treating mumps and hepatitis. It has also been used along with acupuncture and Western medicine to achieve a 90 percent cure rate for encephalitis.

Dosage: 2–3 pills, 3 times per day

Manufacturer: Plum Flower

Warnings and contraindications: It is recommended to avoid brands which use artificial dyes. In any type of infection, seek the help of a health care practitioner.

Chuan Xiong Cha Tiao Wan

Pronunciation and translation: "chwahn shuhng chah tyow wahn"—"ligusticum and green tea pills"

Indications: Headache and nasal congestion due to the common cold

Ingredients:

Mentha haplocalyx herb (Bo He)

Ligusticum wallichii rhizome (Chuan Xiong)

Notopterygium incisium rhizome (Qiang Huo)

Angelica dahurica root (Bai Zhi)

Asarum sieboldi plant (Xi Xin)

Siler divaricata root (Fang Feng)

Schizonepeta tenuifolia herb (Jing Jie)

Glycyrrhiza uralensis root (Gan Cao)

Description: Chuan Xiong Cha Tiao Wan is especially indicated for headaches due to the *wind cold* type of common cold. Typical symptoms are chills, nasal congestion, stiff neck and upper back, and headache, especially in the back of the head (occiput). The chief ingredient in the formula is Ligusticum wallichii (Chuan Xiong), an aromatic herb that is indicated for a variety of headaches, especially those due to *cold*. Notopterygium rhizome (Qiang Huo) is another important ingredient, because it relaxes the upper back and neck when the muscles are contracted from the influence of *cold*. Angelica dahurica (Bai Zhi) and Wild Ginger (Xi Xin) relieve nasal congestion and have an analgesic effect on the head and sinuses. To fight off the cold, the classic combination of Schizonepeta (Jing Jie) and Siler (Fang Feng) is added. Although green tea is included in the name of the formula, it is not one of the ingredients. The traditional way to take this remedy is to wash it down with green tea. This directs the formula's effects to the head and, along with Field Mint (Bo He), adds a cooling effect to moderate the warming herbs in the formula.

Dosage: 8 pills, 3 times per day

Manufacturer: Lanzhou Foci

Warnings and contraindications: Not to be used for *heat*-type headaches, with fever, sore throat, or dry, burning nasal passages.

Er Chen Wan

Pronunciation and translation: "uhr chen wahn"—"two old-medicine pills"

Indications: Excessive phlegm in the lungs and stomach, with symptoms of nausea and cough with abundant clear mucus

Ingredients:

Pinellia ternata rhizome (Ban Xia)
Citrus reticulata peel (Chen Pi)
Poria cocos fungus (Fu Ling)
Glycyrrhiza uralensis root (Gan Cao)

Description: The two "old medicines" referred to in the formula's name are Tangerine peel (Chen Pi) and Pinellia rhizome (Ban Xia). These herbs are highly prized when they have been aged and treated, especially Tangerine peel, which is much more expensive when its aroma is enhanced through aging. Both of these herbs have a drying effect on mucus in the Lungs and Stomach, helping to alleviate coughs or vomiting with large amounts of clear phlegm. The addition of Poria (Fu Ling) and Licorice (Gan Cao) helps to enhance digestive strength (Spleen Qi). This is essential in imbalances involving excess mucus, which is formed when digestive energy is weak. Er Chen Wan manages to treat both the cause and symptoms of this imbalance with a simple four-herb formula.

If the excess mucus is due to the common cold, it is necessary to augment this remedy with a formula that expels the pathogenic influence, such as Chuan Xiong Cha Tiao Wan (see p. 74) or Gan Mao Ling, described below.

Dosage: 8 pills, 3 times per day

Manufacturer: Lanzhou Foci

Warnings and contraindications: This formula has a drying effect, which is why it is indicated for excessive clear, loose phlegm. For this same reason, it should not be used when there is phlegm that is yellow or green and difficult to expectorate. For such a *heat*-type cough, Pinellia Root Teapills (see p. 80) is a more appropriate remedy.

Gan Mao Ling

Pronunciation and translation: "gahn maow ling"—"cold formula"

Indications: Common cold or flu, especially in the early stage

Ingredients:

Ilex pubescens root (Mao Dong Qing)

Isatis tinctoria root (Ban Lan Gen)

Chrysanthemum morifolium flower (Ju Hua)

Vitex rotundifolia fruit (Man Jing Zi)

Lonicera japonica flower (Jin Yin Hua)

Mentha haplocalyx herb (Bo He)

Description: In areas where it is well known, Gan Mao Ling is the remedy of choice when the early symptoms of the common cold arise. When it is taken in the early stage, the cold can often be completely averted. If the symptoms are full blown, it will take longer to work, but the cold will still go away faster than it would without the remedy. Although its ingredients are all cooling, Gan Mao Ling can still be used in *cold*-type illness. In this case, it should be combined with Bi Yan Pian (see p. 71) or Chuan Xiong Cha Tiao Wan (see p. 74). If the cold is accompanied with a severe sore throat or fever, it can be combined with Chuan Xin Lian Pills (see p. 72) or Yin Qiao Jie Du Pian (see p. 81). For stomach flu, it can be taken with Curing Pills (see p. 33) or Huo Xiang Zheng Qi Wan (see p. 29).

Dosage: 4 pills, 3 times per day

Manufacturer: Plum Flower

Warnings and contraindications: It is recommended to use Plum Flower brand, which is free of pharmaceuticals and artificial coloring.

Lo Han Kuo Infusion; Luo Han Guo Chong Ji

Pronunciation and translation: "law hahn gwaw chung jee"—"momordica fruit instant tea"

Indications: Dry, *heat*-type cough, with possible sticky phlegm

Ingredients:
Momordica grosvenori fruit (Luo Han Guo)

Description: Luo Han Guo ("smiling Buddha fruit") is the only herbal ingredient in this instant tea. This exotic fruit is round with a brittle egg-like shell; when cracked open, it reveals a clump of sweet seeds. The overall action is cooling, nourishing and moistening, making it ideal for *dryness* in the lungs with an unproductive dry cough or sticky yellow phlegm. It comes in the form of cubes that can be dissolved in water to make a pleasant-tasting tea. The cubes are 5 percent cane sugar, which contributes to the effect of moistening the lungs. The sweet taste of this remedy makes it especially popular with children.
Dosage: 1 cube dissolved in 1 cup boiling water; drink 1 cup, 2 to 3 times per day
Manufacturer: Luo Han Guo Products Manufactory
Warnings and contraindications: Not for coughs with large amounts of clear phlegm that is easy to expectorate.

Ma Hsing Chih Ke Pien
Pronunciation and translation: "mah shing jih keh pyen"—"ephedra apricot stop cough tablets"
Indications: *Heat*-type cough, bronchitis, or asthma

Ingredients:
Ephedra sinica herb (Ma Huang)
Prunus armeniaca seed (Xing Ren)

Gypsum fibrosum mineral (Shi Gao)
Glycyrrhiza uralensis root (Gan Cao)
Platycodon grandiflorum root (Jie Geng)
Citrus reticulata peel (Chen Pi)
Talcum mineral (Hua Shi)
Honey (Feng Mi)

Description: This patent medicine is a variation of an ancient classic formula. It is indicated for coughs and difficulty breathing due to *heat* in the Lungs, making it useful in treating colds, flu, bronchitis, and asthma. The formula reduces fevers and clears *heat* from the Lungs due to the inclusion of two minerals: Gypsum (Shi Gao) and Talc (Hua Shi). The wheezing and difficulty breathing is resolved with Apricot seed (Xing Ren) and Ephedra (Ma Huang). Although the formula only contains 5 percent Ephedra, it is still considered the chief herb in the formula due to its great strength. Ephedra contains ephedrine, a powerful constituent that relaxes the smooth muscles of the bronchial passages and reduces mucus. This makes it ideal for treating asthma. However, care must be taken when using it, since Ephedra also can raise blood pressure and cause insomnia. For this reason, it is best to use this remedy under the care of a qualified practitioner.

Dosage: 4 pills, 2 to 3 times per day

Manufacturer: Siping Pharmaceutical Works

Warnings and contraindications: Ephedra can raise blood pressure and should not be taken by people with high blood pressure, stroke, or heart disease. Do not exceed recommended dosages. Asthma is a life-threatening condition for many people. While herbal medicine can greatly help in its treatment, it is not wise for asthma sufferers to discard their inhaler. Even if it seems like it is no longer needed, it should be kept in case of emergencies.

Pinellia Root Teapills; Pinellia Expectorant Pills; Qing Qi Hua Tan Wan

Pronunciation and translation: "ching chee hwah tahn wahn"—"clear lung, expel phlegm pills"

Indications: *Heat*-type cough, with yellow or green phlegm that is difficult to expectorate

Ingredients:

Pinellia ternata rhizome (Ban Xia)

Arisaema amurense bile-processed tuber (Dan Nan Xing)

Citrus aurantium immature fruit (Zhi Shi)

Scutellaria baicalensis root (Huang Qin)

Citrus rubrum peel (Ju Hong)

Trichosanthes kirilowii seed (Gua Lou Ren)

Prunus armeniaca seed (Xing Ren)

Poria cocos fungus (Fu Ling)

Description: This is a convenient version of a classic formula with strong expectorant action. It is indicated for a *heat*-type cough, in which the phlegm is sticky, yellow or green, and difficult to expectorate. For this type of cough, the logic is to cool the Lungs, moisten and dislodge the phlegm, and clear it from the Lungs. If this is done quickly, it is possible to prevent the trapped phlegm from progressing into a serious upper respiratory infection like pneumonia.

The ingredients in the formula work together to achieve this goal. Prepared Arisaema tuber (Dan Nan Xing) and Trichosanthis seeds (Gua Lou Ren) break up sticky phlegm due to *heat*. Scutellaria root (Huang Qin) helps fight infection in the Lungs, and Apricot seed (Xing Ren) moistens the Lungs and calms the cough. Citrus peel (Ju Hong) and Poria fungus (Fu Ling) help the Lungs produce less phlegm, and Pinellia rhizome (Ban Xia) eliminates phlegm and acts as an expectorant. Finally, Bitter Orange (Zhi Shi) has a descending action, relieving stagnation in the Lungs caused by the phlegm. The combination of these herbs is a very effective way to treat this uncomfortable condition.

Dosage: 6 pills, 3 times per day

Manufacturer: Lanzhou Foci

Warnings and contraindications: This formula is cooling and moistening, which is why it is indicated for phlegm that is yellow or green and difficult to expectorate. For this same reason, it should not be used when there is excessive clear, loose phlegm. For such a *damp*, *cold*-type cough, Er Chen Wan (see p. 75) is a more appropriate remedy.

Yin Qiao Jie Du Pian; Yin Chiao Chieh Tu Pien

Pronunciation and translation: "yin chaow jyeh doo pyen"—"honeysuckle and forsythia clear-toxin tablets"

Indications: Acute symptoms of *wind heat*-type common cold with sore throat, fever, headache

Ingredients:

Lonicera japonica flower (Jin Yin Hua)

Forsythia suspensa fruit (Lian Qiao)

Arctium lappa fruit (Niu Bang Zi)

Platycodon grandiflorum root (Jie Geng)

Mentha haplocalyx herb (Bo He)

Phragmitis communis rhizome (Lu Gen)

Glycyrrhiza uralensis root (Gan Cao)

Lophatherum gracile herb (Dan Zhu Ye)

Schizonepeta tenuifolia herb (Jing Jie)

Description: Yian Qiao is probably the most commonly used Chinese patent medicine in the United States. It is indicated for the *wind heat*-type of common cold or flu, bronchitis, or tonsillitis. The symptoms are sore throat, headache, thirst, fever, and cough. While it is most effective when taken at the first appearance of symptoms, Yin Qiao can still be used to treat a cold after it has fully manifested.

The formula gets its name from the two chief herbs: Jin *Yin* Hua (Honeysuckle flower) and Lian *Qiao* (Forsythia fruit). These two herbs are often combined to treat *heat*-type flu or colds, since they can efficiently clear *heat* from the body while they fight off the external pathogens that cause the illness. Burdock seed (Niu Bang Zi) and Platycodon root (Jie Geng) are included to relieve the sore throat, Phragmitis rhizome (Lu Gen) stops the cough, and Bamboo leaf (Dan Zhu Ye) alleviates thirst. Finally, Licorice root (Gan Cao) harmonizes all the ingredients in the formula; its anti-inflammatory action also helps soothe the sore throat.

Dosage: 4 tablets (half a vial), 3 times per day

Manufacturer: Plum Flower; Tianjin Drug Manufactory. There are also excellent quality American versions of this remedy, such as those made by Planetary Formulas.

Warnings and contraindications: There are numerous variations on this most popular of all patent medicines. Use caution. Some of the other Chinese blends contain over-the-counter drugs.

Remedies for the Skin

Lian Qiao Bai Du Pian; Lien Chiao Pai Tu Pien
Pronunciation and translation: "lyahn chow bye doo pyen"—"forsythia clear toxins tablets"
Indications: Inflammations and infections of the skin

Ingredients:
Lonicera japonica flower (Jin Yin Hua)
Gardenia jasminoidis fruit (Zhi Zi)
Scutellaria baicalensis root (Huang Qin)
Paeonia rubra root (Chi Shao)
Dictamnus dasycarpus bark (Bai Xian Pi)
Forsythia suspensa fruit (Lian Qiao)
Cryptotympana atrata skin (Chan Tui)
Siler divaricata root (Fang Feng)
Rheum palmatum rhizome (Da Huang)

Description: Lian Qiao Bai Du Pian can be used for almost any type of skin condition, including infections, boils, inflammations, poison oak or ivy, and other allergic skin reactions. Skin rashes and infections are often a result of *heat* in the Blood, with accumulated *dampness* and toxicity. This is addressed by herbs that cool the Blood, such as Red Peony (Chi Shao) and Rhubarb root (Da Huang). To clear toxic *heat*, the formula incorporates Honeysuckle flower (Jin Yin Hua), Forsythia fruit (Lian Qiao), Gardenia fruit (Zhi Zi), and Scutellaria root (Huang Qin). Rashes that come on suddenly or have a tendency to itch and spread are considered to be a form of *wind* in Chinese medicine. This pathogenic influence can be expelled from the body by diaphoretic (sweat-inducing) herbs that have the ability to repel *wind*, such as Dictamnus bark (Bai Xian Pi) and Siler root (Fang Feng). In fact, the name Fang Feng literally means "guard against *wind*."

For poison oak and other *damp* skin rashes, this formula can be taken internally along with external application of another formula, Sai Mei An (see p. 34). Although Sai Mei An is an internal medicine for ulcers, it is also very useful as an external application. Simply empty the contents of one or two capsules into the palm of the hand, drip in a little water to form a paste, and spread it on the rash. This will very quickly stop the itching of poison oak or ivy, and it will also help to dry the *dampness*. This is due to the presence of powdered shells, which have an astringent, drying effect. The itching is relieved by Borneol camphor, which is also cooling.

Skin problems can be eliminated much more efficiently if coffee, sweets, and spicy foods are eliminated from the diet.

Dosage: 4–6 tablets, 3 times per day

Manufacturer: Tianjin Drug Manufactory

Warnings and contraindications: Not to be used during pregnancy. This formula contains rhubarb, which acts as a laxative.

Margarite Acne Pills;
Cai Feng Zhen Zhu An Chuang Wan

Pronunciation and translation: "cheye fuhng jen joo ahn chwahng wahn"—"colorful phoenix pearl hide skin boil pill"

Indications: Acne, skin rashes, hives

Ingredients:

Zostera marina seaweed (Hai Dai)

Lonicera japonica flower (Jin Yin Hua)

Rehmannia glutinosa root (Sheng Di Huang)
Pteria margaritifera pearl (Zhen Zhu)
Bubalis bubalis horn (Shui Niu Jiao)
Bos taurus domesticus gallstone (Niu Huang)

Description: Margarite Acne Pills are a reliable treatment for inflammatory skin conditions such as acne, boils, rashes, and hives. Although skin problems are notoriously difficult to treat, this remedy has a good track record. The chief ingredient is Pearl, or Margarita (Zhen Zhu), a substance with a *cold* energy that clears excess *heat* from the Liver. It is combined with other herbs that have a cooling, anti-inflammatory effect. The formula also includes Water Buffalo horn (Shui Niu Jiao), a cooling agent. This is used to replace the original ingredient of Rhinoceros horn, which comes from an endangered species. Seaweed (Hai Dai) and Rehmannia root (Sheng Di Huang) are also included for their cooling, nourishing effect.

It can be very difficult to cure acne without instituting dietary changes. Coffee, greasy foods, sweets, and excessive spices can all create stagnation and *heat* which will create further skin eruptions. Plenty of fresh water, exercise, and sufficient rest are also essential.

Dosage: 6 pills, 2 times per day

Manufacturer: Plum Flower

Warnings and contraindications: Not to be used during pregnancy. Use only Plum Flower brand. Another brand of the formula contains sophoridane, which is a pharmaceutical.

Remedies for the Urinary Tract

Ba Zheng San
Pronunciation and translation: "bah juhng sahn"—"eight herbs to correct urination"
Indications: Urinary tract infection, urinary tract stones

Ingredients:
Lysimachia christinae herb (Jin Qian Cao)
Phellodendron amurense bark (Huang Bai)
Akebia trifoliata stem (Mu Tong)
Dianthus chinensis herb (Qu Mai)
Polygonum aviculare herb (Bian Xu)
Plantago asiatica seed (Che Qian Zi)
Gardenia jasminoidis fruit (Zhi Zi)
Rheum palmatum rhizome (Da Huang)
Glycyrrhiza uralensis root (Gan Cao)

Description: Ba Zheng San is a standard formula for urinary tract infections. The traditional Chinese diagnostic pattern is "*dampness* and *heat* in the Lower Burner" (or Urinary Bladder). The symptoms are frequent and painful urination, scanty or obstructed flow of urine, pain and distention in the lower abdominal area, and a dry mouth and throat. The tongue will often have a thick yellow coating in the back, which is the area that corresponds to the Urinary Bladder.

The formula contains Lysimachia (Jin Qian Cao), which is a diuretic. It helps eliminate stones from the urinary tract, which is another use for this formula. Other herbs that have an affinity for the urinary tract are Dianthus (Qu Mai), a common ornamental that is easy to grow, and Knotweed (Bian Xu), a weed that is common in North America. Both of these herbs are diuretic and antibacterial, as is Akebia (Mu Tong). Phellodendron bark (Huang Bai) and Gardenia fruit (Zhi Zi) both have the ability to eliminate *dampness* and *heat* from the Urinary Bladder.

When fighting a bladder infection, it is important to maintain an acidic urine pH. This can be done by eating protein with each meal and avoiding sweets. It is also essential to avoid coffee, since it is very irritating to the bladder and makes *heat* conditions worse.

Dosage: 8 pills, 3 times per day

Manufacturer: Plum Flower

Warnings and contraindications: A simple urinary tract infection can sometimes progress to become a serious kidney infection. Be sure to consult your health care practitioner whenever you attempt to self-treat any kind of infection. This remedy is for acute urinary tract infections. A chronic infection often needs to be treated with a different approach, such as nourishing Yin and clearing *heat* with Liu Wei Di Huang Wan (see p. 52) or Zhi Bai Di Huang Wan (see p. 96).

Long Dan Xie Gan Wan

Pronunciation and translation: "luhng dahn shyeh gahn wahn"—"gentian clear the liver pills"

Indications: Urinary tract infection, conjunctivitis, prostatitis

Ingredients:

Gentiana scabra root (Long Dan Cao)

Scutellaria baicalensis root (Huang Qin)

Gardenia jasminoidis fruit (Zhi Zi)

Alisma plantago-aquatica rhizome (Ze Xie)
Plantago asiatica seed (Che Qian Zi)
Akebia trifoliata stem (Mu Tong)
Angelica sinensis root (Dang Gui)
Bupleurum chinense root (Chai Hu)
Rehmannia glutinosa root (Sheng Di Huang)
Glycyrrhiza uralensis root (Gan Cao)

Description: Long Dan Xie Gan Wan is used to treat a wide range of inflammatory conditions in addition to bladder infections. It is most easily understood when considered from an energetic perspective. Deficiency-type conditions require a strengthening or tonification of the body, but for conditions of excess, the proper treatment is clearing or draining. This formula is strictly indicated for excess-type disorders where imbalance consists of an overabundance of internal climates, such as *heat* or *dampness*. Long Dan Xie Gan Wan is specific for the patterns known as *excess heat* or *damp heat* in the Liver and Gall Bladder, with a symptom pattern that includes red eyes, headache, bitter taste in the mouth, irritability, and possible hearing loss. Other symptoms of Lower Burner *damp heat* are dark or cloudy urine, genital itching or swelling, vaginal discharge, and constipation.

Some of the numerous imbalances that can be resolved by this formula can be organized by organ system:
• Eyes: acute conjunctivitis ("pink eye"), corneal ulcers, acute glaucoma, retinitis
• Ears: acute middle ear infection, acute external ear infection
• Urinary: acute urinary tract infection (kidney, bladder, or urethra)

- Reproductive: genital herpes, pelvic inflammatory disease, vaginal discharge, testicular swelling or inflammation, acute prostatitis
- Systemic: migraine, eczema, herpes zoster
- Liver and Gall Bladder: acute hepatitis, acute cholecystitis

Although the above list of medical conditions appears to be random and unrelated, they all share the same traditional energetic diagnosis. For this reason, it is essential to treat the individual's traditional symptom complex, not the Western disease name. Just as a single Chinese diagnostic category can manifest as numerous different Western diseases, a single Western disease can also have a wide range of Chinese diagnoses, depending on the individual's symptoms and constitutional nature. For this reason, it is always wise to consult with a qualified health care practitioner before self-treating with herbal medicine.

Dosage: 8 pills, 3 times per day

Manufacturer: Lanzhou Foci

Warnings and contraindications: A simple urinary tract infection can sometimes progress to become a serious kidney infection. Be sure to consult your health care practitioner before you attempt to self-treat any kind of infection.

Remedies for Women

Chien Chin Chih Tai Wan; Qian Jin Zhi Dai Wan
Pronunciation and translation: "chyen chin chih tie wahn"—"thousand-gold-piece stop leukorrhea pills"
Indications: Leukorrhea (vaginal discharge)

Ingredients:
Angelica sinensis root (Dang Gui)
Atractylodes macrocephala rhizome (Bai Zhu)
Foeniculum vulgare fruit (Xiao Hui Xiang)
Corydalis yanhusuo rhizome (Yan Hu Suo)
Saussurea lappa root (Mu Xiang)
Dipsacus asper root (Xu Duan)
Codonopsis pilosula root (Dang Shen)
Ostrea gigas shell (Mu Li)
Indigofera suffruticosa pigment (Qing Dai)

Description: This is an effective remedy for vaginal discharges or yeast infections. The formula is appropriate for both *heat*-type discharges (dark color, strong smell) or *cold*-type discharges (light color, no smell). The *heat* symptoms can be addressed with Indigo powder (Qing Dai), which is a cooling, detoxifying antibacterial substance. The rest of the formula is tonifying in nature, since vaginal discharges are often due to a deficiency in Spleen Qi (digestive vital energy). When Spleen Qi is weak, *dampness* tends to accumulate, sometimes appearing in the form of a discharge. Chien Chin uses Codonopsis root (Dang Shen), Atractylodes rhizome (Bai Zhu), Fennel seed (Xiao Hui Xiang), and Saussurea root (Mu Xiang) to strengthen the Spleen and eliminate the *damp* environment that leads to the discharge. Oyster shell (Mu Li) is added as an astringent agent to assist in the drying effect. Angelica root (Dang Gui) and Teasel root (Xu Duan) nourish the Blood and the Kidneys and enhance the overall nourishing quality of the remedy. Corydalis rhizome (Yan Hu Suo) promotes blood circulation and alleviates pain.

Dosage: 10 pills, 2 times per day
Manufacturer: Tianjin Drug Manufactory
Warnings and contraindications: If the discharge is dark-colored and has a strong smell, Yu Dai Wan (see p. 95) is more appropriate.

Nu Ke Ba Zhen Wan; Women's Precious Pills
Pronunciation and translation: "noo keh bah jen wahn"—"gynecology eight treasure pills"
Indications: Fatigue, dizziness, anemia, scanty menses, lack of appetite

Ingredients:
Codonopsis pilosula root (Dang Shen)
Poria cocos fungus (Fu Ling)
Atractylodes macrocephala rhizome (Bai Zhu)
Glycyrrhiza uralensis root (Gan Cao)
Angelica sinensis root (Dang Gui)
Paeonia lactiflora root (Bai Shao)
Rehmannia glutinosa prepared root (Shu Di Huang)
Ligusticum wallichii rhizome (Chuan Xiong)

Description: This is the classic formula for deficiency of Qi (vital energy) and Blood. While this condition also occurs in men, it is especially common in women, since they lose blood on a monthly basis during their menstrual cycle. The remedy combines two formulas: one builds vital energy (Qi), and is known as "Four Gentlemen." It consists of Ginseng or Codonopsis, Atractylodes, Poria, and Licorice. The other formula nourishes Blood and is known as "Four Substances." It contains Rehmannia, Peony, Dang Gui, and Ligusticum. When the two formulas are combined, as in this remedy, the result is known as "Eight Treasures" or "Women's Precious."

The reasoning behind this mixing of formulas is classic Chinese herbal logic. Blood is produced in the body through the assimilation of food by the Stomach/Spleen organ complex. When the digestive Qi is strong, more nutrition is assimilated, enabling efficient production of Blood. The "Four Gentlemen" combination contains herbs that strengthen the digestive Qi of the Spleen, thereby indirectly helping the body produce more Blood. At the same time, the "Four Substances" part of the formula directly builds Blood. The combination of the two is an exceptionally effective way to restore normal blood counts.

Interestingly, one of the traditional uses of "Four Substances" is for poor memory induced by deficiency of Blood. A recent clinical study demonstrated that this herbal combination can significantly improve working memory in rats.

Dosage: 8–10 pills, three times per day
Manufacturer: Lanzhou Foci

Tang Kwei Gin

Pronunciation and translation: "dahng gway jin"—"angelica dang gui syrup"
Indications: Fatigue, anemia, scanty menses

Ingredients:

Angelica sinensis root (Dang Gui)

Paeonia lactiflora root (Bai Shao)

Rehmannia glutinosa prepared root (Shu Di Huang)

Ligusticum wallichii rhizome (Chuan Xiong)

Astragalus membranaceus root (Huang Qi)

Codonopsis pilosula root (Dang Shen)

Poria cocos fungus (Fu Ling)

Glycyrrhiza uralensis root (Gan Cao)

Description: Tang Kwei Gin is very similar to Nu Ke Ba Zhen Wan. However, it focuses more on nourishing the Blood, and it contains Astragalus root (Huang Qi), which has a synergistic action with Angelica (Dang Gui) in raising blood counts. This remedy comes in a pleasant-tasting liquid that can be mixed with water or taken by the spoonful. When used in combination with Nu Ke Ba Zhen Wan, the results can be quite dramatic. Cases of anemia and amenorrhea can often be normalized in the course of one or two months. The formula also has a beneficial effect on the immune system, since it contains many immune-enhancing herbs like Astragalus (Huang Qi), Codonopsis (Dang Shen), and Poria (Fu Ling).

Dosage: 1 tablespoon, 3 times per day

Manufacturer: Plum Flower

Warnings and contraindications: Plum Flower is made by Pangaoshou, a G.M.P. factory. It is free of sugar and preservatives.

Xiao Yao Wan

Pronunciation and translation: "shaow yaow wahn"—
"free and easy wanderer pills"

Indications: Premenstrual syndrome with irritability, sore breasts and menstrual imbalances

Ingredients:

Bupleurum chinense root (Chai Hu)

Angelica sinensis root (Dang Gui)

Atractylodes macrocephala rhizome (Bai Zhu)

Paeonia lactiflora root (Bai Shao)

Poria cocos fungus (Fu Ling)

Glycyrrhiza uralensis root (Gan Cao)

Zingiber officinale fresh rhizome (Sheng Jiang)

Mentha haplocalyx herb (Bo He)

Description: This is the standard formula to clear stagnation from the Liver. In traditional Chinese medicine, the Liver ensures the smooth flow of emotions and bodily processes, especially in the reproductive organs. When the vital energy (Qi) of the Liver is stagnant, there can be symptoms of irritability, outbursts of anger, fullness in the chest and abdomen, breast pain, and menstrual irregularity. Xiao Yao Wan soothes and detoxifies the Liver, making it the treatment of choice for pre-menstrual syndrome. A course of treatment takes three to four months, using the formula every day except on the days when there is menstrual bleeding. It successfully treats PMS by eliminating the cause rather than merely suppressing the symptoms.

The chief herb in the formula is Bupleurum root (Chai Hu), which is the primary agent for clearing stagnation from the Liver. It is assisted by Field Mint (Bo He) and

Peony root (Bai Shao), which also act to soothe and nourish the Liver. The formula also contains Atractylodes rhizome (Bai Zhu), which strengthens vital energy, and Angelica sinensis (Dang Gui), which builds Blood and has a regulatory effect on the uterus. Xiao Yao Wan, and all other remedies that treat the Liver, will work best if stress can be reduced and coffee, high-fat foods, and excessive sweets are eliminated from the diet.

Dosage: 8 pills, 3 times per day

Discontinue use during menstrual bleeding. A course of treatment is typically three to four months.

Manufacturer: Lanzhou Foci

Yu Dai Wan

Pronunciation and translation: "yoo dye wahn"—"heal leukorrhea pills"

Indications: Heat-type vaginal discharge

Ingredients:

Rehmannia glutinosa prepared root (Shu Di Huang)
Angelica sinensis root (Dang Gui)
Paeonia lactiflora root (Bai Shao)
Ligusticum wallichii rhizome (Chuan Xiong)
Phellodendron amurense bark (Huang Bai)
Ailanthus altissima root and stem bark (Chun Gen Pi)
Alpinia officinarum carbonized rhizome (Gao Liang Jiang)

Description: Yu Dai Wan is especially useful for *heat*-type vaginal discharges when there is an underlying Blood deficiency. (Chien Chin Chih Tai Wan (see p. 90) can be used for vaginal discharges due to both *heat* and *cold*.) Yu Dai Wan contains a high percentage of Ailanthus bark (Chun Gen Pi), which is astringent and *cold* in nature. When combined with Phellodendron bark (Huang Bai), the two herbs powerfully clear the *heat* and *dampness* that characterize this disorder. The other herbs in the formula nourish the Blood and help alleviate the fatigue and irregular menstrual cycle associated with Blood deficiency.

Dosage: 8 pills, 3 times per day

Manufacturer: Lanzhou Foci

Warnings and contraindications: For a clear-colored vaginal discharge, use Chien Chin Chih Tai Wan (see p. 90).

Zhi Bai Di Huang Wan; Chih Pai Ti Huang Wan

Pronunciation and translation: "jih bye dee hwahng wahn"—"anemarrhena and phellodendron with rehmannia pills"

Indications: Hot flashes, night sweats, irritability, menopausal symptoms, all due to strong *heat* arising from Yin deficiency

Ingredients:

Rehmannia glutinosa prepared root (Shu Di Huang)

Dioscorea opposita root (Shan Yao)

Cornus officinalis fruit (Shan Zhu Yu)

Poria cocos fungus (Fu Ling)

Alisma plantago-aquatica rhizome (Ze Xie)

Paeonia suffruticosa root-bark (Mu Dan Pi)

Phellodendron amurense bark (Huang Bai)

Anemarrhena asphodeloides rhizome (Zhi Mu)

Description: This is a variation of Liu Wei Di Huang Wan (see p. 52), or Rehmannia Six Teapills, previously described in the chapter on tonifying herbs. The name of the formula reflects the addition of two herbs, *Zhi* Mu (Anemarrhena rhizome) and Huang *Bai* (Phellodendron bark). These ingredients enhance the cooling effect of the formula, making it very useful in treating the hot flashes and night sweats that occur in menopause.

Zhi Bai Di Huang Wan treats both the root cause and the symptoms of menopause. The drop in estrogen levels typically reflects a deficiency of Kidney Yin essence. This is replenished with Kidney-nourishing herbs like Rehmannia root (Shu Di Huang), Chinese Yam (Shan Yao), and Dogwood fruit (Shan Zhu Yu). The rest of the ingredients address the *heat* symptoms that are caused by a lack of cooling, moistening Kidney Yin.

Many women have found this formula to be a welcome alternative to hormone replacement therapy, which carries an increased risk for breast cancer.

Dosage: 8 pills, 3 times per day

Manufacturer: Lanzhou Foci

Warnings and contraindications: Rehmannia can be difficult to digest, so this formula should be discontinued if excessive loose stools become a problem.

Products Containing Non-vegetarian Ingredients

Many vegetarians want to avoid medicines made from animals. This is especially true for vegans, who use no animal products at all. Some patent medicines contain shells of sea animals, fossilized bones, insects or shed insect skins, cow's bile, and other animal parts. Others contain endangered species, but none of those products are reviewed in this book. For those who want to make the discrimination, this section lists the patent medicines in this book that contain animal parts. Formulas containing honey, considered by some an animal product, are not included here.

Name of Patent Medicine	Non-vegetarian Ingredients
Chien Chin Chih Tai Wan	Ostrea gigas (oyster shell)
Die Da Zhi Tong Gao (Plaster for Bruise)	Eupolyphaga sinensis (roach insect) Stegodon orientalis (fossilized bone)
Jin Gu Die Shang Wan	Eupolyphaga sinensis (roach insect)
Lian Qiao Bai Du Pian	Cryptotympana atrata (cicada skin)

Margarite Acne Pills	Pteria margaritifera (pearl)
	Bubalis bubalis (water buffalo horn)
	Bos taurus domesticus (ox gallstone)
Ming Mu Di Huang Wan	Haliotis diversicolor (abalone shell)
Pinelia Root Teapills	Arisaema amurense (ox bile-processed tuber)
Sai Mei An	Pteria margaritifera (mother-of-pearl shell)
	Arca inflata (ark shell)
	Cyclina sinensis (clam shell)
Wei Te Ling	Sepia esculenta (cuttlefish bone)

Recommended Reading on Chinese Medicine

Between Heaven and Earth, Harriet Beinfeld & Efrem Korngold, Ballantine Books, New York, NY, 1991.

Chinese Healing Secrets, Bill Schoenbart, Publications International, Lincolnwood, IL, 1997.

Chinese Herbal Cures, Henry Lu, Sterling Publishing, New York, NY, 1991.

Chinese Herbal Patent Formulas, Jake Fratkin, Shya Publications, Santa Fe, NM, 1986.

Chinese Patent Medicines: A Beginner's Guide, Mark Taylor, Global Eyes International Press, Santa Cruz, CA, 1998.

Chinese System of Food Cures, Henry Lu, Sterling Publishing, New York, NY, 1986.

Healing with Chinese Herbs, Lesley Tierra, The Crossing Press, Freedom, CA, 1997.

Healing with Whole Foods, Paul Pitchford, North Atlantic Books, Berkeley, CA, 1995.

Outline Guide to Chinese Herbal Patent Medicines in Pill Form, Margaret Naeser, Boston Chinese Medicine, Boston, MA, 1990.

Planetary Herbology, Michael Tierra, Lotus Press, Santa Fe, NM, 1988.

Plain Talk about Acupuncture, Ellinor Mitchell, Whalehall Inc., New York, NY, 1987.

The Ginsengs, Christopher Hobbs, Botanica Press, Santa Cruz, CA, 1996.

The Healing Power of Ginseng & the Tonic Herbs, Paul Bergner, Prima Publishing, Rocklin, CA, 1996.

The Web That Has No Weaver, Ted Kaptchuk, Congdon & Weed, Chicago, IL, 1983.

Resources

Recommended Sources for Chinese Patent Medicines, Herbs, and Extracts

Botanical Therapy
P.O. Box 1405
Asheville, NC 28802
(800) 447-2066

Botanical Therapy is a small company specializing in concentrated liquid extracts of Chinese formulas. They are known for their fast-acting formulas for insomnia, allergies, tight muscles, and injuries.

Mayway Corporation
1338 Mandela Parkway
Oakland, CA 94607
(510) 208-3113, fax: (510) 208-3069

Mayway Corporation is a very reliable source of Chinese patent medicines. They are especially careful to buy from companies that follow the high cleanliness and quality standards of G. M. P. Mayway also has a full selection of bulk herbs.

Tashi Enterprises / Min Tong Herbs
318 7th Street, #1
Oakland, CA 94607
(800) 538-1333, fax: (800) 875-0798
internet: www.tashi.com

Tashi Enterprises distributes the Min Tong line of concentrated crystal extracts and tablets, which are typically stronger than powdered raw herbs or patent medicines. They are manufactured in Taiwan under pharmaceutical G.M.P. standards. Many of the formulas mentioned in this book are available from them in this form.

Sources of Chinese Herb Seeds and Live Plants

Horizon Herbs
P.O. Box 69
Williams, OR 97544
(541) 846-6704, fax: (541) 846-6233

Horizon grows a variety of Western and Chinese medicinal herbs by organic methods, and their seeds are very reliable. Richo Cech, chief farmer and weed puller, is also very knowledgeable about herbal medicine, and he has written some informative pamphlets on growing and using medicinal herbs.

Richters
Goodwood Ontario, L0C1A0 Canada
(905) 640-6677, fax: (905) 640-6641
email: info@richters.com

Richters has a huge selection of herb seeds and some live plants. They have an expanding selection of Chinese herbs. The live plants ship well, sometimes arriving a little pale and disheveled, but adapting quickly to their new home.

Elixir Botanicals
Brixey, MO 65618
(417) 261-2393

Elixir has a small, but beautiful full-color brochure of their organically grown seeds, with a nice selection of Chinese herbs. The pictures of the mature herbs are really outstanding, and their seeds germinate readily.

Oregon Exotics
1065 Messinger Road
Grants Pass, OR 97527
(541) 846-7578

Oregon Exotics specializes in seeds and live plants of exotic species from around the world, with a good selection of Chinese medicinal species and their relatives.

Newsletters

Healing Fields
P.O. Box 1405
Asheville, NC 28802

Published quarterly, Healing Fields provides information about traditional Chinese medicine, research on herbs, therapeutic dietary recipes, and tips on strengthening the immune system and fighting disease. Cost: $25 per year.

National Organizations for Traditional Chinese Medicine

American Association of Oriental Medicine
433 Front Street
Catasauqua, PA 18032
(610) 266-1433, fax: (610) 264-2768
email: AAOM1@aol.com

The American Association of Oriental Medicine is a national professional association incorporated in Washington D.C. in 1983. It was organized to develop Oriental medicine as a widely acceptable form of complementary medicine. AAOM has become the nation's strongest advocate for national recognition of the Oriental medicine profession as well as serving as a springboard for the creation of the National Commission for the Certification of Acupuncturists. In order to become a member, a practitioner must be a diplomate of the NCCA or have passed the California licensing exam. They will provide referrals to practitioners who are members of their organization. They are also a good source of referrals to practitioners in California, who aren't required to take the NCCA exam and might be missing from that list.

National Acupuncture and Oriental Medicine Alliance
14637 Starr Road SE
Olalla, WA 98359
(206) 851-6896, fax: (206) 851-6883
email: 76143.2061@compuserve.com

The National Alliance is the national professional membership association founded in 1993 to represent the diversity of practitioners of acupuncture and Oriental medicine in the United States. The National Alliance is committed to: fostering high quality health care, education, and research; integrating acupuncture and Oriental medicine into the American health care system; expanding public understanding of the profession; promoting and cultivating discussion, broad representation, and empowerment of members at state, regional, and national levels.

Voting membership is open to practitioners who are state licensed, who are nationally certified by the NCCA, or those who have graduated from an accredited school.

National Certification Commission for Acupuncture and Oriental Medicine (NCCA)
P.O. Box 97075
Washington, DC 20090
(202) 232-1404, fax: (202) 462-6157

The National Commission was established by the profession in 1982 to promote nationally recognized standards of competence for acupuncture and Oriental medicine. They have certified over 7,000 individuals in Acupuncture and 1,000 in Chinese Herbology. NCCA certification is used as the basis for licensure in 90% of the states that have set standards of practice for acupuncture. Certification in acupuncture is based on a candidate's ability to meet eligibility standards of education and/or experience; passage of the comprehensive written and practical examination; successful completion of an NCCA approved course in Clean Needle Technique; and commitment to the professional code of ethics. The NCCA certification program in Chinese Herbology, established in 1994, is now being considered by several states as the basis for licensure to practice Chinese herbology. (California requires proficiency in Herbology as part of their state exam). A new certification program in Oriental Bodywork Therapy was opened in July 1996.

All diplomates undergo a re-certification process every two years. It is based on criteria that reflect competency to practice a healthcare profession, along with continued activity and current knowledge in the field. The NCCA is certified by the National Commission for Certifying Agencies, the agency with the highest voluntary standards of certifying agencies in the U.S.

The NCCA will provide a list of their diplomates upon request.

Schools of Traditional Chinese Medicine

The following is a complete list of schools in North America that specialize in acupuncture and Oriental medicine. To find out information about accreditation, contact the National Accreditation Commission for Schools and Colleges of Acupuncture, 1010 Wayne Avenue, Suite 1270, Silver Spring, MD 20910, phone: (301) 608-9680. The Commission is recognized by the U.S. Department of Education. It is an independent body that establishes accreditation criteria, arranges site visits, evaluates those programs that desire accredited status, and publicly designates those programs that meet the criteria.

Studying to become a practitioner is a challenging, expensive endeavor that will take three to four years of hard work. It is recommended that a prospective student visit some schools and sit in on classes and clinics to get a first-hand impression.

Arizona

Phoenix Institute of Herbal Medicine and Acupuncture
P.O. Box 2659
Scottsdale, AZ 85252

California

Five Branches Institute
200 Seventh Avenue, Suite 115-A
Santa Cruz, CA 95062
(831) 476-9424, fax: (831) 476-8928

Pacific College of Oriental Medicine
7445 Mission Valley Road
San Diego, CA 92108
(619) 574-6909, fax: (619) 574-6641

American College of Traditional Chinese Medicine
455 Arkansas Street
San Francisco, CA 94107
(415) 282-7600, fax: (415) 282-0856

Samra University of Oriental Medicine
600 St. Paul Avenue
Los Angeles, CA 90017
(213) 482-8448, fax: (213) 482-9020
email: 71652.2742@compuserve.com

Emperor's College of Traditional Oriental Medicine
1807-B Wilshire Boulevard
Santa Monica, CA 90403
(310) 453-8300, fax: (310) 829-3838

Royal University of America
1125 W. 6th Street
Los Angeles, CA 90017
(213) 482-6646, fax: (213) 482-6649
email: 73164.3230@compuserve.com

Yo San University
1314 Second Street, Suite 202
Santa Monica, CA 90401
(301) 917-2202, fax: (301) 917-2203

Keim Yung Baylo University
1126 N. Brookhurst Street
Anaheim, CA 92801
(714) 533-1495, fax: (714) 533-6040

Academy of Chinese Culture & Health Sciences
1601 Clay St.
Oakland, CA 94612
(510) 763-7787, fax: (510) 834-8646

American Institute of Oriental Medicine
4683 Mercury Street, #C
San Diego, CA 92111
(619) 467-9890

Meiji College of Oriental Medicine
1426 Fillmore Street, Suite 301
San Francisco, CA 94115
(415) 771-6266, fax: (415) 771-1036

Santa Barbara College of Oriental Medicine
1919 State Street, Suite 204
Santa Barbara, CA 93101
(805) 682-9594, fax: (805) 682-1864

Colorado

Colorado School of Traditional Chinese Medicine
1441 York Street, Suite 302
Denver, CO 80206
(303) 329-6355, fax: (303) 388-8165

Southwest Acupuncture College
6658 Gunpark Drive
Boulder, CO 80301
(303) 581-9955, fax (303) 581-9944

Florida

Academy of Chinese Healing Arts
505 South Orange Avenue
Sarasota, FL 34236
(941) 955-4456

Acupressure / Acupuncture Institute
9835 Sunset Drive
Miami, FL 33173
(305) 595-9500, fax: (305) 595-2622

Florida Institute of Traditional Chinese Medicine
5335 66th Street North
St. Petersburg, FL 33709
(813) 546-6565, fax: (813) 547-0703

National Institute of Oriental Medicine
1724 S. Bumby Avenue
Orlando, FL 32806
(407) 898-8898, fax: (407) 894-0902

Florida Institute of Acupuncture & Midwifery
100 E. Broadway
Oviedo, FL 32762
(407) 366-8615, fax: (407) 366-0145

Sarasota School of Natural Healing Arts
8216 S. Tamiami Trail
Sarasota, FL 34238
(941) 966-7117, fax: (941) 966-4414
email: SSNHA@aol.com

Worsley Institute of Classical Acupuncture
6175 NW 153rd Street, Suite 324
Miami Lakes, FL 33014
(305) 823-7270, fax: (305) 823-6603

Hawaii

Hawaii College of Traditional Oriental Medicine
P.O. Box 457
Kula, HI 96790
(808) 573-0899, fax: (808) 573-2450

Tai Hsuan Foundation College of Acupuncture
2600 S. King Street, #206
Honolulu, HI 96826
(800) 942-4788, fax: (808) 947-1152

University of Health Science
1778 Ala Moana Boulevard, Suite 1307
Honolulu, HI 96815
(808) 951-8242

Massachusetts

New England School of Acupuncture
30 Common Street
Watertown, MA 02172
(617) 926-1788, fax: (617) 924-4167

Maryland

Maryland School of Traditional Chinese Medicine
4641 Montgomery Avenue, Suite 415
Bethesda, MD 20814
(301) 907-8986, fax: (301) 718-0735

Traditional Acupuncture Institute
The American City Building
10227 Wincopin Circle, Suite 100
Columbia, MD 21044
(301) 596-6006, fax: (410) 964-3544

Minnesota

Minnesota Institute of Acupuncture and Herbal Studies
1821 University Avenue, Suite 278-S
St. Paul, MN 55104
(612) 603-0994, fax: (612) 603-0995

New Mexico

International Institute of Chinese Medicine
Rt. 17, Box 52-A
Santa Fe, NM 87505
(800) 377-4561, fax: (505) 473-9279

Southwest Acupuncture College
325 Paseo de Peralta, #500
Santa Fe, NM 87501
(505) 988-3538, fax: (505) 988-5438

New York

The New Center College for Wholistic Health Education
& Research
6801 Jericho Turnpike
Syosset, NY 11791
(800) 922-7337, fax: (516) 364-0989

Pacific Institute of Oriental Medicine
915 Broadway, 3rd Floor
New York, NY 10010
(212) 982-3456, fax: (212) 982-6514

Pymander Acupuncture O.M. Center
121 E. 37th Street, #4B
New York, NY 10016
(203) 227-1715

Tri-State Institute
80 8th Avenue, 4th Floor
New York, NY 10011
(212) 242-2255, fax: (212) 242-2059

Oregon

Oregon College of Oriental Medicine
10525 Cherry Blossom Drive
Portland, OR 97216
(503) 253-3443, fax: (503) 253-2701

Texas

Beijing College of Acupuncture and Oriental Medicine
of Texas
2901 Montgomery Street
Fort Worth, TX 76107
(817) 737-7401, fax: (817) 737-9079

Academy of Oriental Medicine, Austin
2700 W. Anderson Lane, #304
Austin, TX 78757
(512) 454-1188, fax: (512) 454-7001

Texas Institute of Oriental Medicine & Acupuncture
2405 South Shepherd
Houston, TX 77019
(713) 529-8332

Texas Institute of Traditional Chinese Medicine
4005 Manchaca Road
Austin, TX 78704
(800) 252-5088, fax: (512) 444-6345

Washington

Bastyr College of Natural Health Sciences
14500 Juanita Drive, NE
Bothell, WA 98011
(206) 823-1300, fax: (206) 823-6222

Northwest Institute of Acupuncture and Oriental Medicine
1307 N. 45th Street, #300
Seattle, WA 98103
(206) 633-2419, fax: (206) 633-5578

Wisconsin

Midwest Center for the Study of Oriental Medicine
6226 Bankers Road, #8
Racine, WI 53403
(414) 554-2010, fax: (414) 554-7475

Canada

Institute of Traditional Chinese Medicine
368 Dupont Street
Toronto, Canada M5R IV9

Canadian College of Acupuncture
855 Cormorant Street
Victoria, BC
Canada V8W 1R2
(604) 384-2942, fax: (604) 360-2871

59784>

7 42851 00695 3